Don't Diet!

To Chris,

Go for it and have fun!

Fat Loss & Fitness
the Isaac Way

Ric Isaac

Eamon Murphy

The health information in this book is not
intended to replace the advice and supervision
of a qualified health professional.

For further information about
this book, or to order a copy,
phone or fax 08 9438 1199 or
Internet ordering:
www.australian-bookshop-online.com

Isaac, Ric.
Don't Diet! : Fat Loss & Fitness The Isaac Way

First Edition September 2002
Second Printing November 2002

ISBN 0 646 49973 4.

1. Physical fitness. 2. Reducing exercises.
3. Weight loss. I. Murphy, Eamon. II. Title

613.71

Text Copyright © EMRI Press 2002
P.O. Box 1442
Fremantle
Western Australia 6959
Illustrations Copyright © EMRI Press 2002

Printed by Success Print
7a Goongarrie Street
Bayswater
Western Australia

CONTENTS

4

ACKNOWLEDGEMENTS

We wish to thank very deeply the following people who assisted in the research, writing and production of this book.

All the staff of the Sports Science Department of Edith Cowan University, Flora Casotti, Barry Harwood, Deborah Street, Terry Webster, Alyssa Murphy, Ilanna Murphy, Tricia Faughnan, my co-author and whip cracker Eamon Murphy and all of my clients that I have had the pleasure to train and support. You are my teachers as well as my students. You give me the motivation to be the best I can be. Thank you all.

Last but not least my family for always believing in me and giving me the courage to take risks.

Ric Isaac

To Ric for helping change my life. And to Leola, Siobhan, Ilanna, Aislinn and Alyssa for your love and support and for putting up with my obsession and lots of late nights. Special thanks to Alyssa who managed the project from start to finish and who kept me sane and to Jeff Dittrich of Success Print for a thoroughly professional job.

Eamon Murphy

INTRODUCTION

Why another book on fat loss and fitness?

Australia is in the grip of an epidemic – an obesity epidemic. According to the Australian Bureau of Statistics (*Australian Social Trends 1998*), over half of men and women aged over 18 were classified as over fat or obese. What is even more worrying is that obesity among Australian children has doubled in the last 10 years hitting 20%. And Australians are also unfit. Only about 18% of men and 10% of women exercise at a level needed to get minimally fit. If you are worried about carrying excess fat or not being as fit as you would like, you are certainly not alone.

Experts in Australia warn that unless urgent preventative programs are taken, Australia may become the fattest nation in the world in as little as a generation. And this will have enormous consequences for the health system as well as the health and happiness of individuals and their families.

At any time in Australia, about one in four women and about one in six men are trying to lose fat. Most will fail in spite of the warnings of the medical profession, the huge diet industry, which is worth millions of dollars world wide, and the thousands of magazine articles written on dieting. Using many existing approaches to fat loss you have a much better chance of being cured of most cancers than you have of beating obesity.

We wrote this book, therefore, because most people don't know how to effectively lose fat and get fit. They are bombarded with information and are thoroughly confused with the conflicting claims of the various diet "experts". Most diets fail with over 90% of dieters either putting all the fat on again or even getting fatter. And those who fail feel more disempowered, helpless and depressed – and it's not their fault! It's ironic that Australia is the second largest fattest nation on earth when in fact we have some of the world's best experts on nutrition. And in Australia we have easy access to some of the best and cheapest foods in the world and have superb facilities for exercising.

The good news is that we now have many research studies that tell us very clearly how people can lose excess fat by making small lifestyle changes to what they eat and how much they move. The answer to the fat and fitness crisis is ridiculously simple: don't diet, eat better food more often and get more exercise. The evidence is there but you need to dig deep through all the rubbish, conflicting claims and inaccuracies before you find the real facts. And this where our book can help you. We have found the evidence and we provide a simple, safe, scientific approach based on that evidence that has been proven to work.

By using the principles described in this book you will become leaner, fitter, stronger and more flexible. And the benefits will be enormous. You will feel, look and be healthier. Your self-esteem and self-confidence will soar. You will be much less likely to suffer from the diseases associated with our affluent society. Heart and circulatory diseases, diabetes, hypertension, many kinds of cancers, crippling diseases such as osteoporosis, even conditions such as mild depression, can now be prevented and, in some cases cured, by simply leading a healthier lifestyle. Don't just take our word for it. Hard nosed medical scientists say the same thing.

The program we describe in this book – the Isaac Way, developed by co-author Ric Isaac – is very simple. You won't have to count calories, measure portions of food, or join a fat loss program – or ever go hungry. There are no gimmicks. And the program is safe. Your whole family will benefit from following the guidelines. And finally, the program is scientific. It is based on the latest scientific research of nutritionists, exercise physiologists and medical researchers. The program we discuss has worked brilliantly for us as individuals as well as Ric's many clients and we look forward to sharing our information and our experiences with you.

Ric Isaac

Eamon Murphy

1.

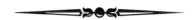

Not another diet book:
The Isaac Way in a nutshell

In this chapter, we introduce you to the fat loss and fitness program that has been developed by co-author Ric Isaac. The key feature of the program - the Isaac Way - is to make small, sustainable changes in four key areas: nutrition, movement/exercise, strength, and flexibility.

We discuss how this book is different from others on fat loss and fitness and why the program works so well. And we will tell you something about our credentials and us. A key feature of the book is that it is based on the latest scientific research on fat loss and fitness so that you will have the right information to make your own choices. While we have tried to make the book as simple and easy to read as possible, it does contain a lot of important information. You may wish to skim read the book before reading in depth. For your convenience we have included key summary points at the end of each chapter. By reading these summaries you will get a very quick overview.

It is most important to understand that you don't have to give up any special foods that you really enjoy, ever go hungry again or take-up an exercise program that causes pain or is unpleasant. The changes that we ask you to consider are gradual and easy. For example, we ask you to consider eating oats instead of wheat-based cereal for breakfast, to walk up the stairs instead of taking the lift or to simply to drink more water. In the following chapters, we will discuss these changes in detail.

For the moment, we will briefly explain each of the four key aspects of the program and the concept of synergy - that is, by getting lots of small things right you will achieve powerful results.

The four key elements of the Isaac Way

Good nutrition

Good nutrition — eating well — is the single most important factor in good health, fat loss and fitness. Eat well for best health! Most Australians do not eat well enough. They do not eat enough of the right foods. Good food provides your body with the nutrients, energy and protection that you need for maximum health. All the other aspects of our program depend upon you getting your nutrition right. In chapter two, we show you how to eat more and better than you have ever eaten before. And never go hungry.

Movement or exercise

One of the most important scientifically proved facts about fat loss is that most people who lose fat and, more importantly, keep it off, have one thing in common: they all exercise. Don't be put off by the word exercise. By exercise, we mean simply moving around more. If you are physically active, you will burn up more fat, have more energy and your body will operate more efficiently. Getting physically fit does not have to involve going jogging or lifting heavy weights. Our motto is "no pain: lots of gain". If you have hated exercise in the past, you will find that the suggestions in chapter three will get you wonderfully fit with minimum effort.

Strength

Being strong means having greater muscle density. The latest research tells us that building up muscle helps greatly in fat loss. Muscles burn fat even when you are resting. In addition, good muscle tone will help prevent aches and pains and enable you to carry out many more daily activities that will burn up fat. In chapter four, we suggest simple ways to become much stronger no matter how tired and/or weak you feel right now. You can build up important muscle strength simply by doing easy exercises at home. You don't have to go to a gym. The best news is you can get stronger whether you are 26, 56 or 86. Remember, increased muscle mass does not mean increased muscle size. Instead, your muscle density will increase giving you more strength, tone and definition without bulk.

Flexibility

Being flexible means that you can move more easily. It also means that your body will be more efficient in burning fat. Flexibility keeps you young and supple. Simple stretch and relaxation exercises that we show you in chapter five will ensure that you are flexible as long as you live. There are other benefits associated with increased flexibility: it can reduce stress which is often a reason why people overeat, it enables you to relax completely, it is fantastic as a toning and strengthening exercise and it increases circulation, promoting toxin release and fat metabolism (fat loss). It is also great as a preventative medicine.

The awesome power of synergy

A key principle in our program is synergy. Synergy simply means that 2 + 2 can equal 5, 6, 7 or more. For example, if you eat well, you have more energy. If you exercise more, you will burn up fat. However, if you combine exercise and good nutrition you will get far greater benefits than if you put a lot of effort into either one. If you combine just a little good nutrition, exercise, strength training and flexibility, you will have a very powerful health package - the Isaac Way.

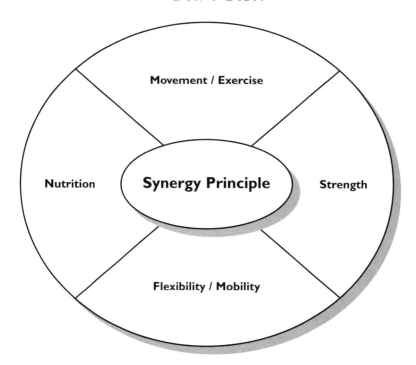

A magic pill for fat loss and fitness?

Imagine for a moment if your doctor were to tell you that a wonderful new pill had appeared on the market that had no side effects and guaranteed the following:

➤ You would lose fat forever while eating well.

➤ You would have much more energy, move easier and have a wonderful feeling of well-being.

➤ Most of your aches and pains that you wake with every morning would either disappear entirely or be greatly diminished.

➤ Your chances of living longer and feeling better into older age would greatly increase.

➤ You would feel younger, stronger and more confident.

➤ Medical problems, including high blood pressure and diabetes, could either disappear or greatly diminish.

➤ Your friends and family would comment on how wonderful you are looking.

➤ You would need a completely new wardrobe and enjoy shopping for clothes again.

➤ You would be better able to make decisions, be more assertive and set achievable goals.

➤ You would cope much better with stress and anxiety.

How much would you pay for such a pill?

The bad news of course is that there is no such pill nor is there likely to be one. Drugs don't make you healthy. At best, they alleviate symptoms. The good news is that you don't need a pill. You can achieve all the above results for absolutely nothing except perhaps for the cost of this book and making some easy changes to your lifestyle.

The wonderful news about fat loss and health gain is that it is never too late to lose fat, get fit and build new muscles. Co-author Eamon Murphy started the program at the age of 64. But he's just a spring chicken. Numerous studies have shown that people in their 70's and older can make very important changes. Nor does it matter how much extra fat you are carrying now. In fact, if you have a serious amount of fat to lose, you can achieve results much quicker once you start this program. Not only will you lose fat faster, but also the hidden strength that your body has developed carrying around the extra fat will be revealed and your energy levels will increase remarkably.

The fat loss was fantastic but the best result of the program was my increased energy levels. I feel alive again - a new woman at the age of 54.

JANET, MELVILLE

We can imagine what you are thinking at this moment. You have heard these promises before so why should you believe us? How is this book different from the thousands of other fat loss books that are published each year?

Not another diet book

This book is different from most other books on fat loss in a number of ways. First, it is not a diet book because diets don't work. Well over 90% of people who lose weight on a diet eventually put all the weight back on again and sometimes more. Instead, the Isaac Way provides a holistic approach that emphasises eating plenty of the right foods and doing some gentle, painless exercise. By holistic we mean that to achieve fat loss, fitness and the ultimate goal of good health one must consider the body as a whole: its need for good food, fitness, strength and flexibility and their relationship with the mind. Most people who go on a diet and do strenuous exercise for weight loss fail because they feel deprived, sore and very tired. And even more importantly because their bodies will rebel. And adopting a holistic approach means that you work <u>with</u> your body rather than trying to fight it.

Dieting makes you fatter

Most popular diet books and weight loss programs appear to be designed to distort people's nutrition and disrupt their metabolism so as to make them fatter and sicker. They are designed to keep people repeatedly coming back to highly profitable and terribly unsuccessful diet programs for the rest of their lives.

SPORTS NUTRITIONIST DR MICHAEL COLGAN

To sum up, this book integrates the scientific knowledge of fat loss and fitness with a program that is sustainable, painless, energising and fun. It shows you how to incorporate the program into your everyday life and gives you the knowledge to succeed. It is about simple but extremely important lifelong lifestyle changes.

In addition, it is the first book that we know of that has been written by an exercise physiologist, Ric Isaac, in collaboration with his client, Eamon Murphy. It provides the insights and the knowledge of both of us. It is therefore both highly practical and solidly scientific. You can take it from us we have discussed, researched and occasionally hotly debated every suggestion and fact in this book for well over 18 months. And we have applied the principles with excellent results in both our lives.

In addition, we don't tell you how much fat you need to lose. We are not in the business of nagging. We wrote the book to provide information so that you as an individual can make your own choice. Some of you reading the book may decide to make large changes to your eating and exercise habits. Others may decide to change just a few things. Yet others may decide they are happy the way that they are – at least for the time being. And that's fine. We've included comments by some of Ric's clients that you may find useful and motivating.

A major reason why most diets and weight reduction programs fail is that somebody else lays down the rules. People are told what they must do rather than making up their own minds. As Dr Rick Kausman, a medical practitioner specialising in weight management and eating behavior puts it, *We need to gather all the relevant information and find the best way of putting it together for each one of us.* We could not agree more. We will give you the latest information and you can decide what you want to do with it. (Dr Kausman's book is in our Reading List.)

About us

We believe in this book because we have, individually and together, thoroughly researched the scientific basis for effective fat loss and for getting fit and we have applied the principles to ourselves with great success, as have Ric's other clients.

Before I met Ric, I had tried many times to lose fat but the diets that I went on eventually failed. Although as a social scientist I'm trained to be critical and to analyse evidence, I became completely lost in the diet jungle. I found much of the information confusing, misleading and contradictory. So when Ric suggested that I try his approach I was initially skeptical and for a long time questioned everything he told me because much of what he said was so contrary to what I had read. For nearly 18 months we've been debating and arguing. I have read the scientific literature extensively to see if I could find a flaw in his methods. But I was not able. I felt strongly that other people should know about his approach - and the best way to achieve this was to write a book together.

EAMON

Ric Isaac is an exercise physiologist and fitness consultant specialising in fat loss. He has a degree in Sports Science, which has provided him with a very solid scientific background in the structure and workings of the human body. He also has diplomas in reflexology and massage, and has studied and taught Yoga for many years. Ric combines mainstream scientific knowledge with alternative strategies. While doing his degree, Ric became interested in the problem of fat loss, especially for older women.

After graduating, Ric worked for two years the Fremantle Leisure Centre as a fitness instructor where he continued to develop his ideas about fat loss and fitness, creating individual programs for both men and women that were highly successful. He is also a qualified Level One Sports Trainer advising elite athletes and training West Australian football umpires. His work experience has added to his theoretical knowledge of exercise physiology, health promotion and nutrition. Ric now runs his own private practice, *Fit for Health*, in Fremantle, Western Australia providing fat loss and fitness programs, reflexology, therapeutic massage, Yoga and nutritional advice.

Ric has worked with men and women of all ages and backgrounds and has helped them become leaner, fitter and happier – as co-author Eamon Murphy can testify.

A university professor, Eamon Murphy has been Ric's client for 18 months. Eamon first met Ric at the Fremantle Leisure Centre and became his client after he had talked to Ric's other clients who were so enthusiastic about Ric's approach. Over 18 months Eamon has experienced dramatic changes to his health and his general well being. He was so enthusiastic that he nagged Ric into writing this book.

By eating more and better quality food and by sensible exercising Eamon has achieved:
- A loss of 10 kilos of body fat.
- A large increase in muscle size, strength and weight.
- An increase in his fitness levels that place him among the top 5 % of 45 year-old males and slightly above average for a 22 year old – not bad for a 64 year old!
- A reduction in his waist size from a potentially dangerous 105 cm to a safe 91 cm.
- A drop in blood pressure to such an extent that he has been able to give up taking hypertension medication after more than twenty years.

THE PROOF

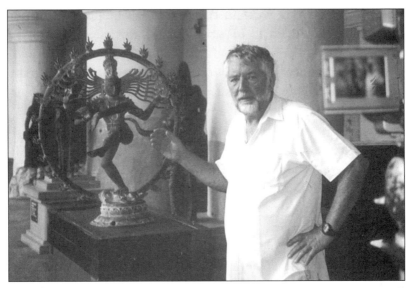

30 Years Dieting

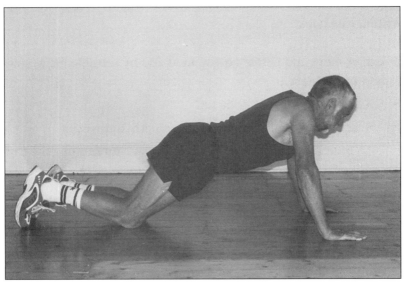

6 Months The Isaac Way

➤   Exceptionally low cholesterol and blood sugar levels.

➤   A rise in energy and enthusiasm for work and play.

➤   Greater self-confidence and self-esteem.

While I was delighted with the fat loss as this was my primary goal, I never anticipated the remarkable benefits to all aspects of my health and life. My only complaint is that I had not read what is in this book 35 years ago.

EAMON, EAST FREMANTLE

Remember, when Eamon began the Isaac Way he was a 64 year-old who had battled fat, at various times in his life, since he was 26. If he can do it, anybody can.

If you are interested in trying the Isaac Way, ask yourself,

Do I really want to lose the excess fat, be fitter and enjoy better health?

Am I prepared to make small changes regularly and build them into my normal lifestyle?

Am I prepared to be patient?

If you answered yes to these three questions then this book can show you how to develop your own strategies for success.

Preparing for success

One of the most important aspects of any change in lifestyle is preparing your mind for success. In her book, *Strong Women Stay Slim*, Dr Miriam Nelson sets out seven secrets for losing fat and gaining fitness. Like any other goal, this requires preparation and planning as well as action. Some suggestions that you may decide to use:

1. Believe that you can do it

Many people have tried to lose fat in the past and failed. As we've said, they failed because they did not know how. The weight loss

industry and our society's obsession with thinness gives us
negative subliminal messages that become translated into negative
self-talk. As a result, we put ourselves down with self-talk. Those
of us who carry excess fat are very familiar with phrases such as:
I haven't got the willpower to do it.

Change your negative affirmations to positive ones. *I am a strong
willed person.* What you believe about yourself has a very
powerful influence on what you do. No matter what has
happened before, trust that you <u>can</u> do it now. This program will
show you how.

2. Take responsibility

Making changes takes time and a little effort. Yet, as mentioned
above, the changes we suggest are relatively easy to make and do
not require much effort. Everyone can be lean and fit. Even so,
change requires that individuals take responsibility for their own
health. Of course if you have serious health problems, we advise
consulting your doctor, preferably a GP specialising in nutrition
and fitness, before starting any new fat loss and fitness program.
You may also want to read other books by qualified dieticians,
personal trainers and books on general health and fitness. (We've
listed some of the best in Further Reading.) Remember, it has to
be your decision. People who succeed at fat loss, like people who
give up smoking, are those who decide to change themselves.

3. Set realistic, achievable and sustainable goals

It's easy to sabotage yourself by setting unrealistic, unattainable
goals. Most people want to lose fat far too quickly. They get
disappointed and give up too soon. One study in the United States
found that a group of women lost an average of 16 kilos in 48
weeks, an average of a kilo every three weeks. The study found
that many were disappointed with this slow loss and yet their

achievement was marvellous. People who have the greatest success in maintaining fat loss are those who lose fat slowly. If you lose just a little fat and become just a little fitter, you will have been successful. Keep it up and you will continue to be successful. Keep in mind that feeling good and having energy are often the greatest rewards.

And keep in mind the difference between achievable and sustainable goals. Anybody can get up at 6 am and walk around the block for 20 minutes – once or twice. But how many people would keep it up - especially on wet, cold mornings?

I simply hate exercising in the morning. I'm still tired and grumpy. But I love an afternoon workout when I'm usually full of beans.

ROGER, THORNLIE

And don't be afraid to set tiny goals. You might simply drink three extra glasses of water a day. Or walk to the shops. Or eat fish instead of meat occasionally. If at the end of the week you have succeeded, then reward yourself. Achieving many small goals regularly can build up to a huge achievement in just a few months.

4. *Keep records*

For many people it is crucial to keep some sort of record of your progress. Studies have shown that people who only kept records of the food that they ate actually lost fat. You need to know exactly what is happening so that you will stay motivated. Keeping a diary about the changes you experience can help to reduce negative self-talk. Without some record of your progress, it's too easy to become critical of your efforts.

The records don't have to be complicated. You might want to take a photograph of yourself when you start and then another a few months later and compare the results. You can simply photocopy one of the menu sheets in the next chapter and keep a list of everything that you eat for a few days. You may decide to write down how much you exercise each week. A useful record-keeping device is to keep a daily diary, briefly noting down any activities and your feelings about them. It's useful to come back to the diary when you experience those inevitable low points when you feel you are getting nowhere.

For me the worst time was the fifth week. I was starting to get fed up and lose confidence. Fortunately I tried on an old pair of trousers and found I could pull in my belt a notch. This motivated me to keep going and 18 months later I'm celebrating my new body and good health every day.

GARY, FREMANTLE

Using your clothes to measure fat loss is a good alternative to inaccurate weighing scales. Notice which notch you use on your belt or pick out a piece of clothing (such as a dress, skirt, jeans, shorts) that is too small and keep trying it on every six to eight weeks. Be patient and it will happen.

5. Make a commitment and write it down

You've already made a commitment by reading this book. You may find it useful to list a few measurable and achievable goals such as:

- *I will change the breakfast cereal I eat for a week*
- *I will fit into that dress in three months*
- *I will start my exercise program after work on Monday*

For many people, writing down their goals will help to commit them further. You might consider writing your commitment in large letters and putting it somewhere you can see it, such as on the fridge door.

6. Plan for success

People are very busy these days. Many people have a job and are raising a family. Planning helps you to do the important things, not just the things that have to be done. For example, you might sit down for half an hour, plan your menu for the whole week, then go out and do your shopping. If you have the right food in the fridge, making healthy food choices becomes even easier and more convenient. Likewise, planning your exercise program might involve rearranging your day to gain extra time or ringing a friend and agreeing to walk together three times a week. The busier you are and the more stress you are experiencing, the more important it is that you plan to do things for yourself.

I like to make a really healthy vegetable pie on Sunday morning. Then during the week when I'm too tired or I can't think of what to cook I can stick a piece of the pie in the microwave.

LOUISE, SOUTH FREMANTLE

7. Learn from mistakes

Studies of top athletes and other successful people reveal they have one thing in common: they learn from their mistakes. Everybody makes mistakes sometimes. If you go off the eating program for a few days, don't beat yourself up. Ask yourself why this happened and then plan so that it is less likely to happen again. Failing at something and being a failure are two entirely different things. Everybody fails at something some time. The secret of success at anything is to keep going and to learn from the experience.

So, it is over to you. We will show you how to make very simple changes in what and how you eat, and how you move and you will get wonderfully powerful results. It's your responsibility. It's your challenge. Nobody can do it but you. But you will get the rewards. We start with the most important aspect: nutrition.   Chapter 2 shows you why good nutrition is so important in any fat loss program and, just as importantly, why it is necessary for a fit and healthy body.

KEY POINTS

Nutrition – the right food for your remarkable body – is the key to good health.

Nutrition combined with a gentle exercise program, including simple strengthening and flexibility exercises, is an extraordinarily powerful combination.

You don't have to go hungry or to exercise hard – in fact by doing so you can defeat your goals.

You can make small changes, which if you keep making them will lead to great results.

You can make dramatic changes and have results that are more rapid if you choose to.

You can still enjoy eating and drinking.

Consider keeping a record of your progress – it will help you to know that the program is working.

The correct information will help you understand why the choices you make are the correct ones.

2.

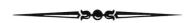

Food, glorious food:
Eating well and getting lean

In this chapter, we explain why good nutrition is so effective for fat loss, fitness and feeling great. However, before you start reading this chapter, you might want to take this simple health quiz to assess your current knowledge about weight loss, diets, nutrition and exercise. You may be surprised by some of the answers.

Health quiz

Answer yes, no or don't know.

1. If you are too fat, is it important to lose weight?

2. Are fats a health hazard?

3. Is good food the most important thing your body needs?

4. Is your doctor the best qualified to give you advice on fat loss?

5. Should you weigh yourself regularly if you are trying to lose fat?

6. Are most diets useless and do they make you fatter?

7. Do reduced fat and low fat products help people lose fat?

8. Is it healthy to lose fat?

9. Is it necessary to exercise to lose fat?

10. Do some foods reduce the risk of getting cancer and other life-threatening diseases?

We will discuss each answer in more detail later. In the meantime, here are some short answers.

1.   If you are too fat, is it important to lose weight?

Not necessarily. Weight loss is not the same as fat loss. For example, most gimmicky diets cause you to lose water and muscle, which you need to help you lose fat.

2.   Are fats a health hazard?

Some fats are a health hazard, but you need good fats to maintain optimal health and promote the metabolism of fats.

3.   Is good food the most important thing your body needs?

Good food is extremely important but you will die very quickly if you don't drink enough fluids. (And, of course, you will die in minutes without oxygen!)

4.   Is your doctor the best qualified to give you advice on fat loss?

Most medical practitioners receive little training in nutrition or fat loss. Some give good advice but others give advice that is either incorrect or confusing. Many concerned GPs refer their clients to nutritionists and other health professionals who specialise in fat loss and fitness. (A useful guide for GPs is Egger, Garry & Binns, Andrew *The Experts' Weight Loss guide for doctors, health professionals ... and to all those serious about their health*. Allen and Unwin, 2001.)

5.   Should you weigh yourself regularly if you are trying to lose fat?

<u>Definitely not!</u> Weighing scales only indicate a loss of weight not a loss of fat. Throw away your weighing scales or, if you have to, weigh yourself once a month.

6.   Are most diets useless and do they make you fatter?

Yes.

7.   Do reduced fat and low fat products help people lose fat?

Not necessarily. Some do, such as skim milk, but many are very high in sugar, which can hinder fat metabolisation.

8.   Is it healthy to lose fat?

Not necessarily. Women in particular can be perfectly healthy if they carry a higher proportion of fat than men. In fact, carrying a higher proportion of fat is necessary for a woman's reproductive system to operate efficiently. However, 'pot bellies' are very much a health risk for men and women. Being too thin is also a health risk.

9.   Is it necessary to exercise to lose fat?

It is possible to lose fat without exercise, but research shows clearly that most people who lose fat and keep it off permanently also do some sort of exercise.

10. Do some foods reduce the risk of getting cancer and other life-threatening diseases?

Yes, especially fresh fruit and vegetables.

How did you go? Many health professionals might miss a few.

Doctors and fat loss

Few doctors feel competent and comfortable in treating obesity. So far obesity has not received much medical attention.

PROFESSOR STEPHAN ROSSER
PRESIDENT OF THE INTERNATIONAL ASSOCIATION
FOR THE STUDY OF OBESITY

10 tips for permanent fat loss

This is the most important section in this book. We strongly urge you to study this section carefully. If you apply most of what we suggest, you will see great improvements in the way that you look and feel. If you don't want to read about the scientific basis for what we say, you may want to skip to the summary of the 10 tips after this section. But we repeat that we do hope that you will study this section very carefully at some time. Knowing the reason for making changes will give you confidence and keep you motivated.

Later in this chapter we will also suggest small changes based on the 10 tips that will make a great difference in how you look and feel.

Tip Number 1 - Drink lots more water

You might be surprised that this tip is the first. It is the first because we consider that drinking enough water is extremely important. For maximum fat loss and good health we urge you to drink at least two litres of water a day (about eight glasses), and preferably 3 to 4 litres, especially if the weather is hot and you are moving around a lot and sweating. You also need more water if you drink coffee or alcohol because they dehydrate you, as does working or travelling in air-conditioning. Hardly anybody in Australia drinks enough water. Few books on nutrition emphasise strongly enough why water is so crucial if you want to lose fat and enjoy great health.

My headaches have stopped completely. I don't know if it's the eating or the drinking water but what a relief to be pain free.

DAVID, NORTH FREMANTLE

The main reason why water is so important for fat loss is that it helps to circulate blood. Blood carries fat, nutrients and oxygen to our working muscles, which increases fat metabolism for energy. Water also helps the de-oxygenated (blue) blood to be pumped back to the heart for more oxygen, nutrients and energy. These fat cells are then carried to the muscles in your body and are burnt up as fuel. Your liver plays a key role in metabolising fat, and it will function much better when water is available to flush out the toxins. So, even if you drink a glass of water before walking down to the local shop, your body will be able to burn more fat.

Drinking lots of water also has many other health benefits besides fat loss:

➤ Water thins your blood and reduces the pressure on your heart therefore lowering your blood pressure.

➤ Drinking water suppresses your appetite.

➤ Your body will be able to quickly and efficiently flush out the toxins (lactic acid) that are created when you exercise.

➤ You are much less likely to suffer from constipation.

➤ For those who suffer from headaches, you may find that drinking more water will cure them.

➤ Because water assists the flow of oxygenated blood to your brain, you will be able to think more creatively.

You can see that water is crucial for feeling your best and for the most efficient functioning of all parts of your body. So cheers! Drink lots of water. Carry around a bottle and sip all day. Have a glass or two when you first get up in the morning. You might fill a container with two or more litres and put it on the kitchen table or your desk at work so you can measure your progress during the day.

Tip Number 2 - Eat lots more fresh fruit and vegetables

Every scientifically based textbook on nutrition stresses the importance of eating a very wide variety of fresh fruit and vegetables. The reason is simple. Our bodies have evolved over millions of years to make most efficient use of unprocessed and unrefined fruit and vegetables. Human beings have spent most of their lives as gatherers and hunters constantly eating a wide variety of natural fruits and vegetables. We still have the bodies of our early ancestors who lived mainly on fruit and vegetables.

Fruit and vegetables provide an excellent supply of the nutrients, vitamins and minerals essential for our bodies to be optimally healthy. The wonderful thing is that you can eat a sackful a day and still lose fat. In addition, fruits and vegetables, along with whole grains and legumes, such as beans and peas, are the best sources of fibre. Fibre is vitally important if you want to lose fat without losing muscle at the same time. Fibre stays in your intestine longer and thus facilitates the slow release of sugars. This will make you less likely to experience mood and energy swings, especially late in the afternoon, when you are most likely to turn to high fat, high sugar snacks. You'll feel fuller and have more energy.

Fibre intake combats heart disease and cancer

The *Journal of the American Heart Association* (October 1999) published a study that found a high intake of fibre not only reduces obesity but also reduces high blood pressure and the risk of heart disease as well as many cancers.

Eating lots of fruit and vegetables may also save your life. Scientists have begun to discover that fresh fruit and vegetables play a key role in protecting our bodies against chronic diseases such as heart disease, diabetes and some cancers. Also you are less likely to suffer from the uncomfortable complaint of constipation. The good news is that you don't have to become a vegetarian to get the benefits of fruit and vegetables. All you have to do is make them an integral part of your daily nutrition.

Eating vegetables protects against cancer

A German study found that vegetarians' natural killer (NK) cell activity was twice as high as meat eaters NK cell activity. NK cells are among the immune system's prime cancer fighting cells. The good news is that you do not need to exclude meat from your diet to gain the benefits. Simply eat more vegetables.

Get into the habit of eating vegetables with as many meals as possible. You can have them as salads, in stir-fries, on open sandwiches, in soups, casseroles, and as snacks. There are many low priced cookbooks available in bookshops and supermarkets that provide tips on how to use vegetables creatively. Of course, you can easily eat fresh fruit at any time.

Aim to eat fruit and vegetables that are in season. These are usually the tastiest and the freshest. If you have access to organically grown fruit and vegetables (that is, produce grown using natural fertilisers without sprays) so much the better, but even packaged frozen vegetables are a good food source. The important thing is to eat lots. And it is much better to eat whole fruit or vegetables that contain fibre rather than juices which do not.

The magic apple

An apple a day keeps the doctor away. Apples, especially apple skins, are high in the antioxidants that help prevent heart disease and certain cancers. A study conducted at the UC Davis School of Medicine in California showed that eating 2 apples or 2 small glasses of 100% apple juice daily for 6 weeks helped reduce the oxidation of 'bad cholesterol' or LDL in the blood. A recent study at Monash University found that eating apples (and other antioxidant rich foods) was associated with less skin wrinkling in a sun-exposed site. A British study reported that men who eat at least five apples a week experience better lung function. To get the most benefits, eat a variety of different apples, particularly those in season.

For more information, see the article "Apples. Do they really keep the doctor away?" in the Monash University medical site: www.healthyeating.com

---

Tip Number 3 - Eat more fish and other sources of good protein

Fish is a super food and Australia has the best fish in the world. We don't eat nearly enough of this wonderfully rich source of protein. Aim to eat fish at least once a day if you can and more often if you want. Fresh fish is best but tinned is fine if it is packed in spring water. Fish provides the protein necessary to build and maintain muscles, skin, bones and blood and, unlike many meats and poultry, fish is very low in fat. If you don't like fish, then you can use other excellent sources of protein such as poultry (free range if you can), nuts, eggs, tofu and other soy products. If you are a vegetarian, increase your intake of nuts, eggs, beans, legumes, pulses, avocado, tofu and other soy products. Just remember not to deep fry.

Fish reduces risk of heart disease

A research team based at the University of Western Australia has shown that you can reduce the risk of coronary heart disease by consuming a small amount of fish each day. The results, published in the American Journal of Clinical Nutrition, show that some fats, such as those found in fish, are important for good heart health.

What about red meat? The experts are divided. A small amount of meat provides useful iron and vitamin B12 as well as being an excellent source of protein. Vegetarians, however, tend to have less body fat and be healthier than meat eaters – which can partly be accounted for by the different lifestyle choices they make. Research has shown that people who don't eat meat tend to have lower blood pressure than those who do. And many meats contain a high proportion of potentially harmful fats. For the case against meat eating you may wish to read John Robbins' *The Food Revolution How Your Diet Can Help Save Your Life and Our World* listed in the Further Reading section of this book. However, most dieticians regard lean meat as a useful food source. We leave the decision to you.

Good protein choices		
Fish grilled/baked	Baked beans	Tofu (firm)
Kidney Beans	Milk (skim)	Tempeh
Lean beef	Yoghurt	Almonds
Eggs	Soy milk	Sunflower seeds
Canned salmon	Peas	Sesame seeds
Tahini	Wheatgerm	Chicken (skinless)
Canned tuna	Avocado	Bean sprouts
Mushrooms	Chick Peas	Lentils

Tip Number 4 - Eat good fats and oils

Because fat is a dirty word in our society we have become fat phobic. Yet, some fats are essential for optimum health and for fat loss. Diets that restrict fat too dramatically are unhealthy and potentially dangerous. The problem with fats is that we eat far too many of the bad ones.

Dieticians, medical researchers and diet experts have been arguing about fat for many years. Some experts advocate a very low fat diet. Others, like the popular but strongly criticised Atkins Diet, advocate large amounts of fat and protein. The debate is very technical and confusing but key facts have now emerged. The following is a summary of the latest research.

Most people in the Western world eat far too much fat, most if it hidden in processed and take away foods. For the majority of us, reducing the amount of fat in our diet will make us healthier and leaner. But having fewer fats does not mean zero fats. If we cut back too much on fat, we will not enjoy excellent health and may, in fact, end up seriously ill. We need to very clearly distinguish between the fats that are good for us and are essential for our health from those fats that make and keep us fat. Most people are very confused because most books and articles, even those written by highly respected authorities, do not make a clear enough distinction between good fats and bad fats.

Eating out and fast foods make you fat

A federal parliamentary report, Cholesterol Levels: Regaining Control! advised restaurants and takeaway outlets to tell their customers how much fat and oils are in their meals. The report blames the industry for the growing cholesterol and obesity problem in Australia. The report stated that all fast-food outlets should display a sign telling customers about the type of oil being used. Representatives from the industry said that it was not their duty and that it would take too much time!

The present reputable scientific consensus is that fats are a very efficient and concentrated source of energy. They help fill us up and make the taste of food more enjoyable. Fats are necessary for healthy skin and hair and contain important vitamins. We need fats to be healthy. The way to ensure that you get sufficient good fats and to achieve optimum health is to eat plenty of the following foods:

➤ fish, especially cold water fish such as salmon, tuna, mackerel and swordfish

➤ nuts, pulses, beans (all kinds)

➤ seeds

➤ very lean meat

➤ poultry (free range if possible)

➤ skim milk, low fat cheese and yogurt

➤ vegetable oils such as extra virgin olive, canola, sunflower or walnut oil in small amounts

➤ soya beans and tofu

You need these to keep healthy and lose fat.

The way to eliminate or cut back on bad (saturated) fats is to avoid the following:

➤ margarine, butter and lard

➤ high-fat meats such as sausages, salami, polony, bacon and prosciutto

➤ chocolate

➤ cakes

➤ processed foods

➤ most restaurant and takeaway foods

➤ products containing coconut, coconut oil and palm oil

➤ full fat cows milk

Beware of labels that contain information such as "containing vegetable fats". Labels like these may indicate that the manufacturer is using cheap, nasty fats. And don't be fooled by processed foods that are labelled "low fat", "low in fat", "97% fat free", "Lite" or "light". A 97 % Fat-Free slice of ham can actually contain 30% of its energy from fat. The confusion has to do with the tricky way manufacturers label their products. Some low fat products are good, but many are very high in sugar and can prevent you from losing fat.

Good nutrition protects against diabetes

A study undertaken at Harvard University School of Public Health published in the Annals of Internal Medicine found that men who ate a lot of red meat, high-fat dairy products and refined flours are 60 percent more likely to develop diabetes from the age of 40. The study recommended that men should increase their intake of whole grains, fruit, vegetables and fish. But obesity remains the most serious risk factor for getting diabetes.

There's no need to be paranoid about fat. We're not saying that you should never eat a piece of chocolate or have fish and chips on the beach on a Saturday night. Just replace the bad fats with the good fats <u>most</u> of the time. Fill your shopping trolley mainly with fresh, unprocessed foods. If you follow the advice of reputable scientifically trained nutritionists, you will not have to worry about fats.

Tip Number 5 - Exercise

Most people will lose fat and, most importantly, keep the fat off if they exercise more. As mentioned above, by exercise we simply mean moving around more often. This may involve simple activities such as strolling around the back garden a few times, kicking a ball with the kids or taking the dog for a walk before work. Walking is an effective, safe exercise, and you don't have to jog or do other vigorous exercise unless you want to. In fact, exercising too hard can stop you losing fat. Remember, no pain means lots of gain.

Exercise is such an important aspect of losing fat that we discuss it in detail in the next chapter.

Tip Number 6 - Get stronger

The latest scientific research shows that simple strengthening exercises that you can do in your own home will build muscles that burn fat even when you are watching cricket or sleeping. We show you how to do these exercises in Chapter Four. When combined with regular exercise and good nutrition, strength training is a powerful way to lose fat and become extremely healthy. Increased strength makes everyday activities such as lifting fun, quick and easy!

Tip Number 7 - Eat five to six times a day

Contrary to most diet advice in the last 30 years or so, it's good to snack. It's more than good - it's extremely important to eat often.

Never go more than three hours without eating if you want to burn fat effectively. Here is why.

By eating more often, your metabolism - the rate at which your body burns energy - is elevated. By eating regularly, you tell your body that there is plenty of food available. When you go hungry, your body thinks that famine is just around the corner. Because humans throughout millions of years of evolution never had enough to eat, the human body has adapted to become extremely efficient at preserving energy. If you don't eat enough, your body simply stops burning fat. Fat is a very precious source of energy, and your body starts consuming carbohydrates or your muscle rather than depleting the reserve of fat in storage. If you starve yourself for long enough, you may die of heart failure as your body eats away at your heart muscles.

But if you eat regularly and frequently, your body has a regular source of energy in the food you are eating and in any excess body fat. This slow release of energy means you will not be tempted to have a high fat snack, cake or alcoholic drink, which you will crave if your blood sugar is low. You will have more energy and be able to move around more and this in turn will burn up more fat. Also, the act of eating burns up fat by working your jaw muscles and fuelling the metabolic process occurring in your stomach (digestion). And eating more meals that are regular can ease digestion and reflux by promoting small and more regular releases of bile by the liver and pancreas.

I get to eat as much as I like! I love it and the fat just slips off!
KAREN, FREMANTLE

Another benefit of eating more often is that after a while you will not eat so much because gradually your stomach will shrink. You will enjoy your food much more, but you will be more quickly satisfied.   You will become more of a gourmet, one who appreciates good food, rather that a gourmand, one who eats too much.

And please make time for the most important meal of the day: breakfast. As the name suggests, breakfast means breaking the long fast that you have been on since the night before. A good breakfast of slow burning foods such as oats / oatmeal with fresh fruit will provide energy for the rest of the day. By eating a good breakfast, you won't experience cravings caused by low blood sugar mid-morning when you may be tempted to have a cake or other unhealthy snack. Eating breakfast will also allow your brain to get a regular supply of nourishment and you will think more clearly and be more productive. Avoid most breakfast cereals as the majority are nutritionally lacking. Not only are they bad for your metabolism, brainpower and hunger pangs but also bad for your purse/wallet.

Tip Number 8 - Never diet

As we have said before, not only do diets not help you lose fat, but they also make you fatter in the long term. This point is so important that we are going to repeat it.   Diets cause many Australians to gain even more body fat. One of the reasons why so many Australians, especially women, are too fat is because they diet. By diet, we mean restricting your intake of food in order to try to lose weight in a short period of time. You know such diets by the advertising: "phenomenal results", "lose ten kilos in two weeks", "secret ingredients", "instant results", "magic herbs that strip fat".

These diets often offer a pseudo-scientific backing such as "laboratory tested", "scientifically proven", "recommended by doctors". The diets that promise miracle results in a short time through sticking to a rigid eating plan are usually far too low in nourishment. These diets include the Soup Diet, the Beverly Hills Diet, the Grapefruit Diet and the Israeli Army Diet.

Getting off the diet treadmill was such a great relief. I've stopped seeing food as something bad and enjoy eating food because I know how much good it's doing me.

ELIZABETH, WHITE GUM VALLEY

Other diets are potentially dangerous because they eliminate or drastically cut back on essential sources of nourishment, for example, the Atkins Diet.

Here's an example of a typical shonky weight loss product taken from the Internet:

> **Lose 1 - Pound Per Day ... Doctor Recommended**
> **Discover How You Can Lose Up to 1 - Pound Per Day,**
> **and Keep it Off ... Permanently!**
> **Only $1.33 Per Day**
> **FREE Doctor Support**
> **Order Today and Receive $397.00 worth of FREE Bonuses!**

The way these claims can be made is that people going on such a diet will initially lose water and muscle but the price they will pay is more than $1.33 per day. They will eventually get very tired, hungry and often sick. Most of all they become dispirited when the "poundage" stops coming off and they go back to old eating patterns. This means that they gain the weight that they lost whilst on the diet plus some more because the body's metabolism has gone into famine mode and is converting food into fat, storing as much as possible to sustain itself through the next 'famine'.

Because the word diet has such a negative image, we prefer to use the term good nutrition which is a lifelong approach to good eating and thus good health.

Tip Number 9 - Throw away your weighing scales

This tip might surprise you. Consider putting your weighing scales in the rubbish bin because they really are a health hazard. We have become obsessive about our weight and yet weight loss – as distinct from fat loss – is not significant or important for good health. The weight and height charts calculated by insurance companies and used by many doctors are very inaccurate. They don't tell you how much fat you are carrying and therefore can be very misleading. For example, on the current height and weight charts a very muscular 35-year-old man may be overweight on the scales but carry no excess fat. Another man of the same height and age may be underweight on the scales but carry a very high percentage of body fat.

It is correct that you will probably lose weight as you lose fat, but by weighing yourself too often you can easily sabotage your fat loss efforts. For most people, the amount of fat they can lose really effectively is about one to three kilograms a month, yet many people want to lose more than a kilogram a week, which cannot be done safely. For example, if you gain muscle, you will weigh more, but as we have seen, muscle burns fat and you will be leaner if not necessarily lighter.

The other point to remember is that your weight varies from day-to-day. For example, if you sweat a lot and don't drink enough water, the scales would show that you have lost a kilogram or two in weight, but all you've really lost is water. If you keep the weighing scales in your bathroom, it is very hard to resist the temptation to see what you weigh. Then if you get what seems like a bad result, you are tempted to do something foolish such as cutting back on food or giving up entirely. One of the best ways to gauge if you are losing fat is to try on clothes that have been tight. If they are loose, you've lost fat no matter what the scales may say.

Having weighing scales in the house also encourages children, especially girls, to become weight obsessive and to develop unhealthy and often dangerous eating habits.

For years my mood each morning was determined by the weighing scales. If I found that I had lost some weight my husband and kids could relax and enjoy breakfast. But next day when the weight had come back on I was devastated and the family would run for cover. It started to become ridiculous. I would weigh myself two or even three times a day. I would find ways of getting the best results such as placing the scales in a different position on the floor or by leaning backwards. It took courage to throw away the scales, but I'm much happier and my family enjoy breakfast every morning.

LYDIA, NORTH FREMANTLE

Tip Number 10 - Reduce or eliminate alcohol - perhaps

This is a tricky one. You can lose fat and enjoy alcohol. If you want to have a drink or two with your evening meal at home or at your favourite restaurant, then fine. Because your body treats alcohol as a poison, your liver works to eliminate it immediately. But alcohol becomes a problem if you eat fats when you drink. If you drink alcohol and eat a high-fat meal, such as sausages or chips or fatty snacks, the fat will be immediately deposited in your body.

Alcohol also provides some energy so if you want to lose fat relatively quickly, you will achieve better results if you eliminate it altogether or restrict it to one day a week. Most experts recommend that you have some alcohol free days each week to give your liver a chance to recover.

There is some good news for those of you who like a drink or two. Research has shown that a small amount of alcohol, particularly red wine, is good for most people, and people who drink very moderately are generally healthier than those who don't drink at all or who drink too much.

The French paradox: drinking red wine is good for you

The French have a relatively low rate of heart disease despite the fact that they eat relatively high levels of unhealthy, saturated fats. It seems they get some protection because many are regular moderate red wine drinkers. One explanation is that red wine contains antioxidants that mop up free radicals that damage the cardiovascular system and other parts of the body. People who drink about one or two glasses of wine a day seem to have raised protection, particularly if they drink with their food. For those of you who don't drink alcohol, you can also get benefits from de-alcoholised red wine or grape juice. Green tea also seems to protect, but white wine and other alcoholic drinks are not so effective.

You might want to photocopy the ten tips and put them somewhere that you can see them every day.

10 TIPS FOR PERMANENT FAT LOSS

1. Drink lots of water.

2. Eat lots more of different kinds of fresh fruit and vegetables.

3. Eat more fish and other sources of good protein.

4. Eat good fats and oils.

5. Exercise – move around more.

6. Get stronger.

7. Eat five to six times a day.

8. Never diet.

9. Throw away your weighing scales.

10. Consider reducing or eliminating alcohol.

Putting the 10 tips into action

Avoid anything that contains lots of bad fats, simple carbohydrates, empty calories and sugars such as:

➢ White and wholemeal bread

➢ Deep-fried foods

➢ Margarine and butter

➢ Most takeaway foods

➤ Most processed, packaged and tinned foods

➤ Ice cream, cakes, biscuits, chocolate and other snack foods

➤ Soft drinks, fruit drinks and "health" drinks such as Gatorade

➤ Full cream cheese, milk and other dairy products

➤ Deep-fried fish and chips

➤ Sausages and other high fat meat products

➤ Toasted muesli and most breakfast cereals

➤ Flour and bread crumbs

➤ Alcohol. If you cannot eliminate alcohol entirely, consider drinking mid-strength beer instead of regular beer or mixing spirits with low-calorie mixers and wine with soda

➤ White rice

For maximum fat loss, reduce or eliminate simple carbohydrates such as:

➤ Wholegrain bread

➤ Bananas

➤ Potatoes

➤ Pasta (all types)

➤ Dried fruit (any)

➤ Brown rice

➤ Fresh fruit juice

(We discuss below the reasons why these foods inhibit fat loss.)

For maximum fat loss eat the following:

➤ Grilled, steamed, microwaved or baked food

➤ Skim milk, ricotta and cottage cheeses

➤ High-quality breakfast cereal such as rolled or quick oats (hot or cold with soy or rice milk), porridge, homemade (not toasted) muesli

➤ Boiled, microwaved, baked foods

➤ Fresh fruit

➤ Fresh vegetables – eat as much as you want

➤ Fish (tinned or fresh)

➤ Chicken, eggs, nuts, tofu, tempeh and other soya products

➤ Hommous

➤ Beans, grains and legumes such as millet, corn, rye, chickpeas, lentils and sunflower seeds

➤ Lean meat (perhaps)

The debate over simple carbohydrates and fat loss

For most effective fat loss, limit or avoid simple carbohydrates such as bread, rice, pasta, most cereals (except oats), potatoes, bananas, dried fruit and fruit juices. Many reputable dieticians in the past have recommended these foods, but the latest research suggests that fat loss will become more difficult if you eat them. If you are close to your ideal body size or exercising very heavily, then simple carbohydrates are fine although they are not essential for good health.

I used to eat loads of bread and pasta in the evening, but when I cut them out I noticed how quickly I started to lose fat. Now that I am close to my ideal size, I enjoy a couple of slices of bread each day and a potato in the evening.

TOM, EAST FREMANTLE

There are two main reasons why simple carbohydrates are not ideal for fat loss.

Simple carbohydrates, such as white bread, are quickly turned into blood sugar, which prevents your body from burning fat, the alternative energy source. Human evolution over millions of years has taught your body to conserve fat in case of famine which was always just around the corner. If simple carbohydrates are available, your body will simply not burn fat. In addition, simple carbohydrates provide only short bursts of energy leaving you flat and tired when they are quickly burned up. Imagine simple carbohydrates as a piece of brightly burning paper that is quickly consumed, but complex carbohydrates as a smouldering log that provides a steady supply of energy for a long time.

I used to eat two rounds of sandwiches for lunch and would start to nod off in the afternoon. I now eat just one piece of bread but lots of fish and salad and have much more energy.

OSCAR, BEACONSFIELD

Secondly, simple carbohydrates don't provide enough of the essential vitamins, minerals and protein and that we need to function optimally. Consequently, when we 'fill up' on bread or pasta we physically can't eat enough of the nutrient rich foods that our body needs to function effectively.

If we provide our body with complex carbohydrates (listed below), our metabolism will convert stored body fat into energy and all our body systems will function more effectively.

There are also important differences between simple carbohydrate foods. Brown rice is a better choice than white rice. Heavy grainy breads are better than white or wholemeal, while wholemeal pasta is better than white pasta. But best of all are the complex carbohydrates listed below which release slowly into the blood stream providing steady, long term energy.

Good carbohydrate choices

Vegetables (raw)	Vegetables & pulses (cooked)	Fruits (fresh/canned)
Alfalfa sprouts	Artichoke	Apple
Bamboo shoots	Asparagus	Apricots
Broccoli	Beans, green	Blackberries
Cabbage	Bok choy	Blueberries
Capsicum	Broccoli	Cantaloupe
Cauliflower	Brussel sprouts	Cherries
Celery	Cabbage	Grapefruit
Cucumber	Cauliflower	Grapes
Endive	Chick peas	Kiwifruit
Lettuce	Eggplant	Lemon
Mushrooms	Kidney beans	Lime
Onions	Leeks	Mandarin
Radishes	Lentils	Nectarine
Snow peas	Silverbeet	Peach
Spinach	Spinach	Pear
	Yellow squash	Pineapple
	Zucchini	Strawberries
		Watermelon

I can't believe how easy it is! Now that I know what and when to eat my body fat has dropped amazingly.

JULIE, EAST FREMANTLE

18 simple ways to better eating

Instead of having two sandwiches, have an open slice of bread with lots of filling.

Instead of eating a large serving of pasta, add some extra vegetables and cut back on the pasta.

Replace your meat or chicken with fish.

Have low fat or skim milk instead of full cream milk.

If you have to eat fast food, eat lunch at Subway (lots of salads and skip the dressings) instead of fast food stores.

Have a glass of wine instead of beer or a spirit and mixer.

Eat nuts instead of chocolate for a snack.

Drink a glass of water instead of a can of soft drink.

Grill your fish, chicken or meat instead of deep-frying.

Eat sweet potato or pumpkin instead of potato.

Pack your own lunch with lots of fruit and vegetables instead of buying sandwiches or pies.

Cut back on most foods that are labelled "light", "lite", "fat reduced", "97% percent fat free" but are often high in sugar.

If you normally have three vegetables in a dish, add two more and have less of the filler such as rice, bread or pasta.

When you eat out, have a large salad as an entree.

Use hommous or avocado as a spread rather than butter or margarine.

Eat heavy, grainy breads such as soy and linseed instead of white or wholemeal.

Have a vegetarian meal occasionally.

For a snack have home made muesli instead of cake or biscuits.

Develop your own eating plan.

You might like to take a few minutes to work out your own menu using the template on the next page. Make out a shopping list and buy all the ingredients for the week so that each meal will be covered.

You may wish to photocopy your menu and stick it on your fridge to help you keep track of your daily intake. Notice that there is a free day when you eat whatever you wish.

Chapter Six contains some suggestions about developing a maintenance program once you are happy with your fitness level and body shape.

KEY POINTS

Good nutrition – eating the right amount of the right foods – is the single most important factor in losing weight, being healthy and enjoying life.

The most effective way for most people to improve their nutrition is to make small, sustainable changes in what and when they eat.

You may wish to make dramatic changes if you want rapid results, but this will require greater commitment and dedication.

The simplest and most effective way to improve your nutrition is to gradually replace processed foods with fresh foods and drink lots and lots of water.

Eat a wide variety of foods, never skip a meal and never, ever diet.

Eat often – at least five times a day – but have smaller serves.

Enjoy your food and have a day off once a week eating and drinking whatever you want.

EATING PLAN

	Day 1	Day 2	Day 3	Day 4	Day 5	Day 6	Day 7
Breakfast							
Snack							
Lunch							**FREE DAY**
Snack							
Dinner							
Snack (If necessary)							

3

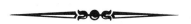

No pain, all gain:
Exercising and getting fit and lean

In this chapter, we want to explain why exercise is so important for getting fit and getting lean. Understanding the relationship between exercise and fat loss is crucial to the success of any fat loss program. We explain why the three major elements of our exercise program, that is, exercise, strength training and flexibility, are so important. By reading this chapter carefully, you will understand better how your body responds to different kinds of movement and, most importantly, how those responses will help to burn fat even when you are asleep or watching the telly with your feet up.

One thing common to almost all people who lose fat - and, more importantly, keep the fat off - is that they build movement and exercise into their daily lives. Scientists are now beginning to find that exercise is a far more important factor in fat loss than medical researchers and GPs once thought. People who exercise regularly not only live longer but also enjoy life much more. They are more energetic, productive and happy.

> ### The great diet debate
> *On February 24, 2000 many of America's best-known nutritionists, doctors and other medical experts met to find out what was the best way to lose fat. At the end of the marathon session the experts could only agree on two things: Americans are too fat and exercise is good for you! If the medical experts are confused it's hardly surprising if you – and your doctors – are bewildered about the best way to lose fat.*

We keep stressing throughout this book the principle of synergy: combining nutrition with exercise, strength training and flexibility. You can lose fat just by exercising alone, but it involves a lot of time and much effort. However, by combining exercise with good nutrition the fat loss is greatly accelerated and involves less physical effort.

The secrets of effective exercise

As we have mentioned before, by exercise we mean just moving your body, not pounding the pavements covered in sweat. Effective exercise is the key because if done correctly, exercise burns energy, which is obtained from fat. So regular amounts of moderate exercise when combined with a good nutrition program will burn off your excess fat more effectively than merely jogging for an hour once or twice a week.

But the benefits go well beyond just the burning of fat while you are exercising. Moderate exercise can also improve your resting metabolism - that is, how fast your body burns energy (calories) when you are not active. As your metabolism increases, you burn fat even when you are sitting in front of the TV or sleeping. Scientists now understand that the increase in metabolism may last for up to 24 hours after you have stopped exercising.

So what does the term 'resting metabolism' mean? Imagine your body as a car engine. When your resting metabolism rises through exercise it is like your car engine idling at a faster rate and thus burning more fuel, or in our case, body fat. It doesn't take that much exercise or movement to make a big difference to fat loss, to your resting metabolism and to how you feel. You don't have to take up vigorous jogging or join an expensive gym. What is really important is that you exercise at a level that is best for you. Exercise, like all other aspects of fat loss and good health, is a highly individual affair. One reader might find that she needs a five mile jog before she feels happy, while another might get enough exercise by walking around the block a couple of times. Fitness levels differ greatly from person to person. Doing the activity and doing it at the right level for you is the key here.

All physical activity counts for fat loss and fitness whether it is incidental and unplanned, such as hanging out the washing, or planned, like walking around the local park with your friend. Another interesting fact is that the more you exercise (providing that you don't over-do it) the more energy you have. And the more energy you have, the more likely you are to exercise because you feel more energetic. And so the cycle goes on.

Unfortunately, many people have had a negative experience with exercise early in life, often in school. It's very sad that many people have been turned off exercise for life because of the emphasis in the past on team sports, winning and on rewarding the natural athletes. This often meant that the good athletes, those who least needed the exercise, got the most exercise and benefits while those who needed the exercise most spent their time bored on the sidelines. Or else peers and sometimes teachers humiliated the unfit because they could not keep up with the others. As a result, many people think that exercise is not for them. They are wrong.

I hated sport at school. But now I am much fitter than many of the sport stars that I used to envy so much.

PAUL, PALMYRA

The good news for non-athletes is that you don't have to be good at sport to be superbly fit. You can become fitter than you have ever been in your life, just like the 65 year old co-author of this book. And you don't have to worry about not being good at sports when you were younger because you can't store fitness, as many former champion sports people discover when they stop heavy training. Look how many former football stars are prime candidates for heart attacks. The human body has a remarkable ability to recover and to grow if you give it a chance. It's never too late to get huge benefits from exercise even if you have never done any planned exercise in your life.

Exercise is so simple even for a 54 year old woman - and I never knew it could be so much fun!

JOYCE, FREMANTLE

Besides its role in fat loss, exercise has been proven to have a much wider range of positive benefits than was previously thought. Research from around the world now shows that exercise plays a key role in preventative medicine. For example, a major study found that exercise, combined with good nutrition, could prevent diabetes. Once you develop diabetes you have it for life and you have to control it through diet, medication or insulin injections. One study found that about 30 minutes of exercise five times a week when combined with healthy nutrition can reduce the incidence of diabetes of those already at risk by 58 %. Adults over 60 years reduced their risk by 71 %.

Weight bearing exercises, such as walking, also help prevent osteoporosis – a fragile bone disease that cripples many older people and forces them out of their homes and into nursing homes. Even a small amount of regular exercise will help protect you against a wide range of other diseases including stroke, heart disease, colon and breast cancers, hypertension and chronic mild depression. Appropriate exercise improves our self-confidence, and thus our self-esteem, and enhances the quality of decision making and creativity. As you can see, besides burning more fat, regular exercise has a huge range of extra benefits - not least is that it slows down the ageing process.

> **Being fit helps you live longer**
>
> *An eight year study on 32,000 men and women of all ages conducted at the Cooper Institute for Aerobics Research, Dallas, Texas found that the big difference between those who died (690) and those who survived was fitness. Even the people who were fat but fit had much lower mortality rates than those who were lean but unfit.*

The quickest way to increase your fitness and to facilitate the most effective loss of body fat without strain is through monitoring your heart rate. Your heart rate tells you if you are training correctly. The easiest way to judge your correct training heart rate is to take the "talk test". Most people exercise too hard when trying to lose fat. You should be able to have a conversation comfortably while exercising. If you can't talk, then slow down. You are working too hard and are sabotaging your progress. But if you can sing lustily or discuss politics without drawing a single breath, then you may need to exercise just a little harder.

I used to go hell-for-leather at all of my exercise classes – really dripping with sweat and exhausted. By slowing down I burned off fat more quickly.

ALEX, EAST FREMANTLE

Here's the scientific explanation for why you should take it easy when exercising.

Your body needs oxygen to burn fat effectively. This occurs during moderate (aerobic) exercise when your body has a good supply of oxygen which it draws upon to metabolise your fat cells and to use them for fuel (energy). But if you are puffing and panting whilst exercising, you are exercising anaerobically and your body tends to burn carbohydrates, which provides a quick source of energy, rather than fat. So no pain really does mean a lot of gain. Exercise at an appropriate level to maximize your fat loss.

Of course, if you want to get very fit, you will need some harder exercise, but if your main goal is to burn fat, then remember the "talk test". The key point to remember is that when oxygen is available, your body burns mainly fat for the energy it needs. Fat provides much more energy than carbohydrates.

The other point to keep in mind is that the fitter you are the more easily your body can oxidise fat even if you exercise hard. In other words, when you first start exercising your body will find it harder to use the fats. But as you get fitter – as you quickly will – your body will become more efficient at burning fat even when you are exercising slightly harder. So when you first start exercising keep the level of intensity right down.

To sum up: very hard exercise uses only carbohydrates and the muscles' stored energy for fuel. Easy exercise means that the body draws upon fat as well as carbohydrates. The lesson is obvious: the less intense the exercise the more fat is used and the leaner you will get. You can, of course, always combine harder exercise to improve your cardio-vascular fitness with some easier exercise to burn fat but, for most people, the first priority will be fat loss.

Monitor your heart rate

The "talk test" is one way to measure whether you are exercising at the right intensity. There are, however, more accurate ways. You can be your own sports scientist. The very simple technique of taking your pulse can help you maintain just the right amount of exercise to burn fat. The correct way to take your pulse is to bend your right arm and hold your hand out palm up. Put two fingers on your wrist in line with the base of the thumb. Press lightly and you will feel your pulse. (If you can't get a pulse you are not doing it correctly - or you are dead!) Count the number of beats over sixty seconds, or count the beats for fifteen seconds and multiply the number of beats by 4. Then check with the table below to make sure you are exercising at the right intensity level.

Another way to measure your heart rate is to use a heart-rate monitor. If you like gadgets and measurements, you might want to invest in one. They are very simple to use. You just strap a band around your chest and a special kind of watch to your wrist. When you turn on the watch you get an instantaneous readout of your heart rate. You can also set an alarm for minimum and maximum heart rates. Basic heart rate monitors cost round $150 and are available in sports stores. Some fancy ones even have a built-in memory that stores your information, which you can then feed into your computer if you are so inclined. You can even print off graphs showing your progress if you want to bore your friends.

I like to use a heart monitor because I tend to go too hard. The monitor reminds me to slow down.

MAX, THORNLIE

Some people find heart rate monitors highly motivating. Others get bored with them very quickly. It's really a personal choice. The main thing is to actually do the exercise. As long as you can take your pulse or do the "talk test" you have all that you need to keep within your target heart rate.

Target heart rate

To lose the maximum amount of fat, aim to keep your heart rate between 50% and 70% of your maximum heart rate adjusted for age. See the table below. If you are very unfit, then simply reduce the heart rate by five to ten beats per minute. Very fit individuals can increase their target heart rate by five to ten beats per minute.

Target Heart Rates in Beats Per Minute (BPM)

Age	20	25	30	35	40	45	50	55	60	65	70	75	80	85	90
BPM	145	141	138	134	131	126	121	117	113	109	105	101	97	92	88

Water and exercise

As we discussed in the chapter on nutrition, very few people drink enough water. If you are exercising you need to drink at least three to four litres a day. Drink lots of water before, during and after exercise - especially during hot weather. Marathon runners know that if they drink enough water, they can substantially reduce their times.

When you think about it, it's no wonder that water is a miracle drink. Water thins your blood and makes your heart and lungs work more efficiently. It helps dissipate the heat that is generated during exercise. It flushes out the toxins (lactic acid) that are generated when you exercise and from everyday life. Water is particularly important for fat loss during exercise because it helps your circulatory system absorb fat cells into the blood stream and transport them to the working muscles, where the fat is used as fuel. Without enough water your body simply can't burn the fat it wants to, so give it all the help it needs. The message is very clear: drink lots of water.

Here are some suggestions for building exercise into your daily routine (and remember you don't have to do a great deal to experience the benefits):

➢ Include both planned (regular walking) and incidental (using the stairs).

➢ Exercise does not have to be planned. Move around as often as you can.

➢ Spread your exercise over the day if you find it easier.

➤ Short (say 10 minute) exercise periods four times a day are just as effective in fat loss and fitness as one continuous 40 minute bout. Many people who start to exercise after a long period of inactivity find the shorter periods much easier to handle.

Start slowly and easily

For many people, slow easy exercise, such as walking, is more enjoyable and more easily built into a daily routine than other more "formal" types of exercise.

Have fun

Find an exercise or exercises that you enjoy and that you can build into a new daily routine. If you like to walk, then walk. You may, for example, take your dog for a walk every evening or if you don't have a dog, walk with your partner or a friend. You may prefer to spend half an hour on the treadmill at your local gym. The more fun you have the more likely you will be to keep it up.

Keep at it!

You may find that the first few weeks of exercise are the hard ones. It takes a little time before you start to feel the benefits, but when you do you will be much more motivated. If you get into a routine, such as going for a walk before dinner, you will be more likely to stick at it. It's sad that so many people stop their exercise program just when they are about to get a huge jump in fitness. It takes about four weeks before a new routine becomes fixed and a similar time to feel the benefits of the increased exercise. That's why regular testing is so important.

After about six weeks on my new exercise and eating program I started to get discouraged because I felt that I was not making much progress. But when I had an assessment I saw that I had made very good progress and this knowledge kept me motivated.

MAYA, FREMANTLE

Be flexible

It's not a great idea to turn exercise into another stressor in your life. If you happen to miss a day or a few days exercise, don't worry. You may even feel better if you have a break. Your body occasionally needs a rest. In fact, if you were feeling ill, a rest would be the best thing for you. The really important thing is to start again - perhaps at a lower level - when you feel better.

Do different kinds of exercise

Cross training, that is doing different types of exercise, has at least two advantages. First, you get to work different groups of muscles. For example if you walk, you will strengthen your legs. If the next day you decide to have a swim, your arms will also get a good work out. Exercising different muscle groups also means that you are less likely to get injured. Second, many people find that doing different exercises stops them from getting bored.

Exercise with a friend or partner

It's a lot more fun for some people to exercise with a regular companion. It's also much more difficult to miss a session when you know somebody else is depending on you to turn up. For instance, you might consider taking up group classes or social sports.

Measure your progress

An easy way to measure your improved fitness is to walk for nine minutes at an easy pace and note how far you have walked. Do this every four weeks at the same place and compare times and how you felt at the start, middle and end. Taking your pulse before and after will increase the accuracy of the test. You will know you have increased your fitness when you can walk the same distance in a shorter time using the same level of effort with a similar or reduced heart rate.

Good gyms and fitness centres can provide a more scientific record of your physical fitness.

20 easy ways to get more incidental exercise

Take the stairs instead of the lift wherever you go.

Walk instead of driving to the local shop.

Ride a bike to work.

Go for a walk before dinner.

Clean your own car instead of having somebody else do it.

Go for a walk during your lunch break.

Trade in your power mower for a hand mower.

Spend more time mucking about in the garden.

Take up a new sport or hobby such as kayaking, dancing or gardening.

Walk around the golf course instead of sitting in a buggy.

Put a bit more effort into cleaning the house.

Get an active dog and take it for a walk.

Carry the shopping bags to the car and always take a carry basket if possible.

Use your cleaning, such as vacuuming and mopping, as an exercise. Do the dishes vigorously.

Play and run with your own or someone else's kids.

Do some muscle tightening and strengthening whilst watching TV.

Go for bushwalks.

Join an exercise group or social sports team.

Park your car or bike five minutes walk away from work, school or the supermarket.

Buy a simple timer, get up and stretch every hour on the hour.

The advantages and disadvantages of different forms of exercise

Exercise	Advantages	Disadvantages
Walking	The safest, easiest and best form of exercise for most people. Can easily be fitted into the normal day. Is very effective. Does not cost anything except perhaps a good pair of walking shoes.	Some people find it boring, especially the hyperactive. More time consuming than some other forms of exercise. Not so efficient for very fit people. May be difficult for a very obese person or those with joint or muscle problems.
Jogging	It can be a highly efficient way of burning energy and getting fit. Can achieve a lot in a short time. Many people find jogging highly addictive as it releases endorphins, which gives the jogger a high. Many people find the social side of jogging with friends to be a very powerful motivator.	Can be very dangerous for those who are very unfit or over fat. Can lead to injuries especially to the knee, ankle or foot. Many – possibly most – joggers exercise too hard and therefore don't burn fat. Some people find jogging unpleasant and boring. Jogging in very hot weather can be dangerous and uncomfortable.
Swimming	Particularly suitable for people who are carrying a lot of extra body fat or those with leg injuries as there is very little stress on the joints and muscles. A great summer exercise. Very few injuries. Ironically benefits most those with poor swimming technique. Swimming is great when you are starting but you might want to incorporate other exercises when you get a bit fitter.	Sometimes inconvenient to get to the pool or the beach. Requires commitment on a cold day. Can be too easy, especially for those who are good swimmers. Because body weight is easily supported in water swimming is less effective than walking for burning fat.
Aerobics	Many people enjoy the music and the social support of exercising to music with an instructor. Fun if done in the right group with the right instructor.	An inexperienced or too enthusiastic instructor can push some members of the class too hard. Some people might be working too hard while others might be taking it too easy. Some aerobic classes attract the "beautiful people" with their flashy gear, which can be off-putting to others.
Cycling	Enjoyable for many people. Weight is supported so less chance of impact injury.	Can be difficult for beginners and larger people. Can be dangerous on busy roads.
Exercise Bikes and Exercise Treadmills	Very easy to monitor progress by programming speed and time. Many have inbuilt heart monitors. Out of the rain, wind, cold and heat. Appeals especially to individuals who like to carefully monitor their programs.	Many people find them boring. Removes some of the fun and spontaneity. Routines can become too rigid. Cost can be high. Most people who buy exercise equipment stop using it after a few workouts.

Warning: train – don't strain. Exercise can be a health hazard

Just because some exercise is good for you doesn't mean that lots is much better. In fact, it can easily set you back. For some people, exercise becomes so addictive that they push themselves into exhaustion, injuries and illness – even death in some cases. In particular, some men, who should know better - like the authors of this book - sometimes leave their brains behind when they start enjoying exercise too much. Highly trained, superbly fit athletes, such as marathon runners, are often very unhealthy because their immune systems are so depressed. Athletes who over train often become what is known as "stale" and take months to recover from tiredness and illness if they push too much. If you exercise too hard your body will not be able to grow and build.

Marathon running is not healthy

A study of 2300 marathon runners found that runners who ran the marathon had six times the instance of colds and influenza when compared to those who decided at the last minute not to run. The moral of this story is that while moderate exercise is good for you, too much exercise can damage your immune system and make you sick. If you are sick, you can't do any exercise and you'll quickly lose your fitness and put on fat – even trained marathon runners.

Some signs that you are over-doing the exercise

➣   You are always feeling tired. Exercise should make you feel much more energetic most of the time - not leave you exhausted.

➣   You get lots of colds and flus. A clear warning that your immune system is under stress.

➣   You are tired and irritable a lot of the time.

➣   You get upset and worried if you have to miss an exercise session. A sign that you are becoming too addicted.

➤ You keep dropping off to sleep during the day but find it hard to sleep at night.

➤ Your resting pulse is elevated. As you get fitter your resting pulse, which you can take first thing when you wake up, will gradually drop. A higher than normal pulse (80 instead of 50 - 70 beats per minute for example) shows that you are not recovering from your exercise.

What is the cure for over-exercising?

Easy! Slow down or take a break.

Good news for big people

People who carry too much body fat have very strong, well developed muscles, especially in their calves and thighs. Carrying around this extra weight builds strong muscles.

If you are now carrying a lot of extra body fat, you have a head start over many slim people who may have very little muscle development. Combining nutrition, flexibility, cardiovascular exercise and strength training provides very rapid results for those carrying a very large amount of extra fat.

Ric constantly reinforces this in his classes by reminding people just how strong and capable they are. Doing squat exercises, for example, is more beneficial for a 110 kg person than a 80 kg individual doing the same exercise. In addition, the bigger person is stronger and has more muscle mass and therefore they burn more fat and get even stronger and fitter.

KEY POINTS

The most common characteristic of people who lose fat and maintain fat loss is that they build exercise into their daily lifestyle.

Anybody of any age or size can benefit hugely from exercise. In fact, the more body fat you carry and the more unfit you are, the more you will benefit from even a small amount of very easy exercise.

To obtain maximum fat loss and fitness you need to work at your ideal training heart rate.

The simplest and most effective indicator of an effective heart rate is to do the "talk test" when you can talk but not sing while exercising.

Exercise can be either planned (going to a gym) or incidental (using the stairs at work). Both forms are very valuable.

Exercise can be either long (30 minutes) or broken into short periods (3 lots of ten minutes) over the day.

Regular assessment of your fitness through the simple measurement of your pulse will help keep you motivated.

Medical research has shown that even a small amount of regular exercise will help protect you against a wide range of diseases including diabetes, stroke, heart disease, colon and breast cancers, hypertension, osteoporosis and chronic mild depression.

Pain does not mean gain and unfortunately most people either do no exercise or exercise far too hard and therefore deny themselves the greatest benefits.

4

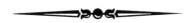

Getting strong and getting lean:
How to burn more fat even when asleep

How would you like to have an inbuilt mechanism that will burn fat even when you are sleeping or sitting watching TV?

The secret is a simple strength training program that is guaranteed to build your muscles and increase your strength whether you are 19 or 90.

You're never too old for strength training

As part of a research project, six women and four men in a nursing home in the USA volunteered to undergo a simple strength training program. The volunteers ranged in age from 86 to 96. Four had serious chronic diseases, including heart disease, diabetes and osteoporosis. The results, which were published in the prestigious Journal of the American Medical Association in 1990, were startling. In just eight weeks, the very frail men and women increased their strength by an average of 175 percent. They also greatly improved their walking speed and balance. Two of the group actually discarded their canes.

Strength training is the third component of our holistic approach to fat loss and fitness. It is also known as resistance training or weight training. The most recent scientific research has shown that strength training is extremely effective in fat loss and in getting and staying healthy, particularly when combined with a good nutrition program and cardio-vascular fitness. The American Heart Association is now telling both doctors and the public that just 20 minutes of weight training two or three times a week can lead to a healthier heart and a longer, more active life. And strength training has numerous other benefits in addition to fat loss.

Anybody can benefit hugely from some strength training. Some of the most exciting research being done in the area of strength training is by Dr Miriam Nelson, a prominent American medical researcher and author of *Strong Women Stay Young*. Dr Nelson found that she was able to increase the strength and quality of life of patients in nursing homes using a simple process of strength training. She was delighted to find that her patients also lost fat as their strength increased. What also surprised Dr Nelson was how quickly her patients gained strength. Within a mere eight weeks women in her study had actually doubled the weights they could lift.

If you think that you are too old to start strength training, you might keep in mind that Dr Nelson worked with patients who were in their 70s and 80s, some with serious medical conditions, and who had never strength trained before. If you are a woman worried about building huge muscles, you can't. To build big muscles you would need to spend hours and hours in the gym or take the hormone testosterone, which stimulates bone and muscle growth. Instead of building huge muscles like a man, you will tone your body with healthy lean muscle.

I lived in fear. Every day I was scared to death of dropping a tea cup or a plate. I didn't trust what little strength I had. Now I relish reaching for the top shelf to bring down a heavy book. I'm much stronger and more confident. As a 71 year old woman I find my new strength amazing.

GRACE, FREMANTLE

You don't even have to join an expensive gym, buy expensive equipment or spend a lot of time. We will show you seven very simple exercises that you can do in your own home that will get you strong very quickly. To get the maximum benefit all you need to invest is 30 - 60 minutes three times a week. However, you will get positive results from even 20 minutes twice a week.

If you want to put more time or spend more money on strength training, we will also advise on a range of options that you may consider such as joining a gym, hiring a personal trainer or buying strength training equipment.

Why build muscle?

One of the most important reasons for building muscle is that muscle burns fat. Muscle requires energy just to maintain itself. It gets its energy partly from the fat in your body. It follows, therefore, that the more muscle you have, the more fat you will burn right around the clock whether you are eating, sleeping or working. By increasing your muscle mass, you will increase your body's ability to burn even more fat as a fuel source. As a further bonus, you will burn more fat when exercising. The muscle story gets even better.

I had read somewhere years ago that we lose muscle as we age so I was resigned to getting weaker as I neared 70. But much to my surprise and delight I found that after a few months of weight training I had larger, stronger muscles than I had thirty years ago. To be honest it gave my ego a huge boost!

KARL, WHITE GUM VALLEY

More muscle mass increases your metabolic rate, which simply means the speed at which your body works and burns calories, including fat. Fat, on the other hand, uses hardly any energy and just sits there slowing your body down. The extra muscle burns more fat and with more energy you can exercise more and build more muscle. Muscle tissue makes your body work faster and more efficiently. But people who go on crash diets lose muscle mass.

Beating osteoporosis – the silent thief

Osteoporosis is called the silent thief because it eats away bone mass gradually over many years. Often the first sign of this bone thinning is when the person breaks a hip or other limb. One of the reasons for the growth of this crippling disease that now affects about 50% of women over 50 is that we no longer lift as many heavy objects as we used to in the past. Prevention? The best way is to strengthen your skeleton and supporting muscles by lifting weights two or three times a week. Regularly climbing stairs, walking up hills and jogging will also help.

Gaining greater muscle strength helps you do everyday activities, such as climbing stairs, shopping, social sport or housework, more easily. It gives you more energy and improves your balance and co-ordination. Having a strong, lean, healthy body will increase self-esteem, self-confidence and decision-making. It will also help you handle stress and depression much better. It strengthens your heart by increasing your cardiovascular fitness especially if you also do some aerobic exercise. And it prevents bone loss, bone fractures and osteoporosis, which is extremely important as you get older. Having a lean, healthy body can reduce blood pressure as well as reduce the risk of heart disease and adult onset diabetes. It can also reduce the symptoms of Parkinson's disease and arthritis, particularly when used in conjunction with a holistic health program of good nutrition, cardiovascular exercise and flexibility.

Things that were a struggle (shopping, washing and cleaning) are now so easy. I can't wait to go shopping to buy my lovely food.

SASKIA, BEACONSFIELD

As we can see, an hour or two a week doing strength training is a tiny investment that will have a dramatic impact on the quality of your life, particularly as you get older.

How to build muscle

The two key factors in strength training are good nutrition and a strength training program that is suitable for you.

We keep emphasising throughout this book the key importance of nutrition. Without good nutrition even the best strength training program would have limited results. But with a well-tailored individualized nutrition program, you will find that your strength will increase dramatically within a few weeks. In order for your muscles to grow most effectively, they need high-quality protein, which you can get in the form of fish, fish oil, nuts, tofu and other soya products, lean high-quality meat and chicken, free range if you can. Be particularly careful about your protein if you are a vegetarian or elderly. Beans, cheese, legumes, eggs (especially the whites), avocado and Bragg's amino acids are all useful protein sources for vegetarians.

Should I buy home gym equipment?

Think carefully before you do. We suggest that you perhaps try out the equipment in the shop before buying it. Some of the equipment is quite useless and unnecessary. Keep in mind also that the salespeople may know nothing about the equipment. Get as much information as you can. It is essential that you receive proper instruction in how to use the equipment properly in order to prevent injury and to maximise benefits.

Should I join a gym?

I tried going to a gym but got bored very quickly. It seemed like too much hard work for me. I prefer more casual exercise that I know I'll stick at because I enjoy it.

ANNIE, FREMANTLE

Perhaps. Some people find that the gym is enjoyable and motivating. You may find new friends and have a great time when you are there. A gym provides access to a wide range of equipment and often a swimming pool. The best also provide regular assessment of your progress. However, be warned! Some gyms make their money out of those clients who only come in a few times. Once they get your money they don't want to see you again until it's time to renew your membership. Some are filled with muscle heads and lycra clad body beautifuls, and you may feel uncomfortable and unwelcome if you don't fit the image. Increasingly however gyms, especially community gyms, are catering for the unfit and older clients and you are just as likely to find a 70 year old working out alongside a 20 year old and nobody noticing.

It is really important to find a gym instructor who really knows what he or she is doing and who can develop a program that works best for you. Using weights can cause injuries so you definitely need proper instruction.

I love going to the gym. I need the discipline and routine and I enjoy the company. I go three times a week at the same time and nothing gets in the way - ever. It's my time.

CLAIRE, BEACONSFIELD

Before deciding to join a gym, ask to look around. You might decide to pay a daily fee before you pay for an expensive year's membership. Enquire whether the gym provides regular assessments (at least every three months) to measure your progress. Find out what qualifications the instructors have. Ask what ongoing support the gym provides. For example, you need to change your program every two months or sooner because your body gets used to the training and the program becomes boring. You need to have the support of a qualified instructor who can give you good, healthy advice.

I feel like a weight has been lifted off my shoulders. My posture and strength have improved enormously. I used to feel like an old man at the age of 61 but now I can't wait to get up tomorrow!

DRAGO, FREMANTLE

Should I employ a personal trainer?

A personal trainer that is right for you can be a great investment. The trainer can take time to assess your health and your level of fitness and then work out the very best program for you. A trainer can also show you how to use gym equipment properly. A good trainer will assess you as a total person and advise you on the best nutrition, cardiovascular exercises, strength training and flexibility exercises. You should be able to call on the trainer when you have difficulties.

But please note that personal trainers in Australia do not need any formal qualifications. Some are young and inexperienced and may well push you far too hard, especially those who do not have a proper background in nutrition and exercise physiology. Probably the best way to find out if the trainer is any good is to ask to see their qualifications and the names of other clients so you can check with them. A good trainer will have a list of clients who have agreed to act as referees.

Most personal trainers charge around $40 to $70 an hour but you may only need a couple of hours to get going and sharing the cost with a friend makes the whole process more economical. We suggest that you read what we have written in this chapter and write down some questions that you could ask of a personal trainer.

Should I keep records?

Yes, if you can. Most people find that a record of improvement is highly motivating. Keep an exercise diary, which can be as detailed or as simple as you like. Reputable gyms and fitness trainers will include a regular physical assessment as part of their service.

7 Strength exercises

On the following pages, we show you 7 simple strength exercises that will increase your strength in all the major muscle groups of your body. Increasing muscle strength will increase your body's ability to burn fat.

The following simple exercises that you can do at home without expensive equipment will build up all the major muscles of the body.

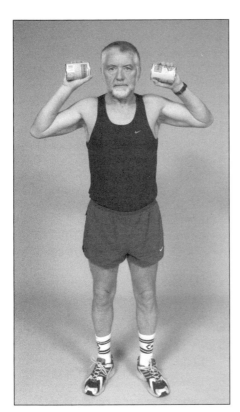
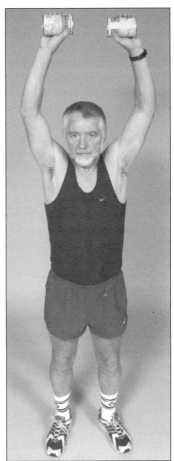

Shoulder press (shoulder and neck muscles): 3 sets of 8 repetitions

Start with your feet shoulder width apart and your arms bent, with the palms of your hands facing forwards.

Keep your wrists locked and the weights close to your ears.

Breathe out as you push your arms up taking them straight above your head and straightening the elbows as much as possible.

Bring the weights together at the top of the movement.

Breathe in as you lower your arms back to the starting position, with the weights next to your ears.

Repeat procedure

Tip: go slower to make it harder. use tins of beans or tomatoes etc as weights and keep buying heavier tins to make it harder as you increase your strength.

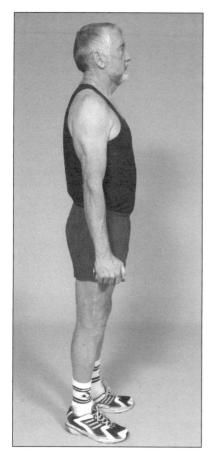 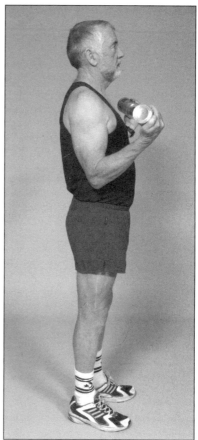

Bicep curls (upper arm at the front): 3 sets of 8 repetitions

Start with your feet shoulder width apart, your arms slightly bent, with the palms of your hands facing each other.

Keep your upper arm by the side of your body the whole way through the movement (only the lower arm moves in this exercise).

Breathe out as you raise your lower arms.

Add a half twist to your wrists so your palms are facing the ceiling as you squeeze up.

Do not allow any movement in the upper arms!

Breathe in as you go down, again twisting the wrist as you lower your arms.

Keep the tension on the muscle by keeping your arms slightly bent.

Repeat procedure.

Tip: Every two weeks use heavier weights to keep getting stronger. Do not let your back sway. Stay upright throughout the whole movement.

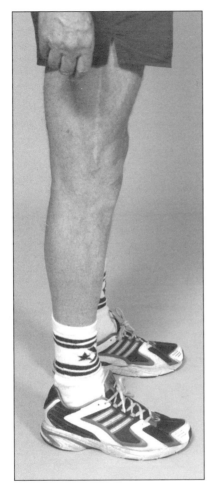 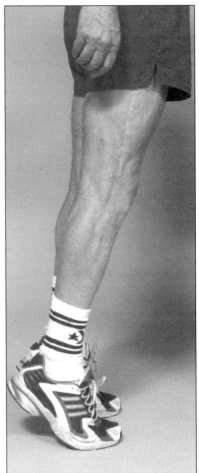

Calf raises (front and back of lower legs): 3 sets of 8 repetitions

Start with your feet shoulder width apart and your legs perfectly straight.

Stand next to a wall so you can balance yourself.

Push up onto your toes breathing out as you go up. Push up as high as you can go.

Keep your legs straight the whole time.

Breathe in as you come down but don't let your heels touch the ground. Keep the tension on the back of your lower legs.

Repeat – breathing out as you push up.

Tip: to make it harder hold at the top for a second or two. Do it on a step with just your toes on the step and your heels hanging free.

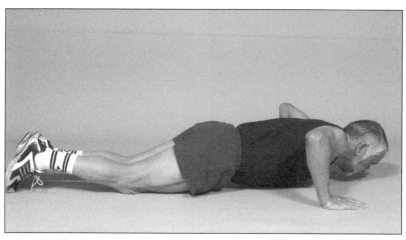

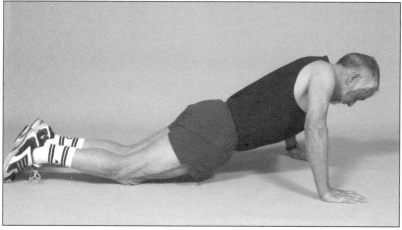

Push ups (chest and back of arms): 3 sets of 8 repetitions

Start on your stomach with your knees slightly bent. Hands are wide apart so your forearms point straight up towards the ceiling.

Keep your eyes on the floor the whole way through the movement.

Breathe out as you push up keeping your pelvis in line with your back. Don't let your buttocks push out!

Straighten your arms.

Then breathe in as you go down bending your elbows at right angles and repeat. Don't let your chest touch the ground.

Tip: to make it easier go down half way. To make it harder go lower and touch the tip of your nose to the floor.

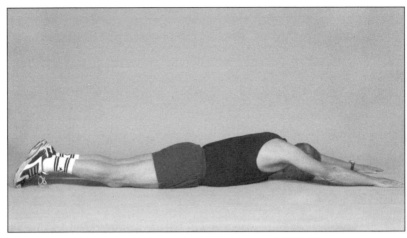

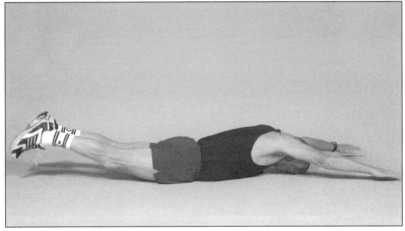

Super person (lower back and buttock muscles): 3 x 15 seconds

Start on your stomach with your arms and legs stretched out. Rest your forehead on the mat/carpet.

Squeeze your thighs, buttocks and stomach muscles and breathe in as you raise your arms and legs a couple of centimetres off the ground.

Breathe in and out as you hold this position.

Remember to keep your forehead resting on the mat.

Think about your buttock muscles and squeeze, squeeze, squeeze!

Tip: to make it easier leave your hands on the floor and just raise your legs. To make it harder point your toes, keep your legs straight and take your arms and legs off the mat/carpet. Gradually increase the time you hold this for.

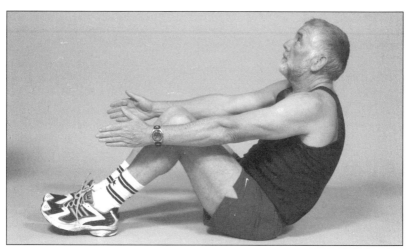

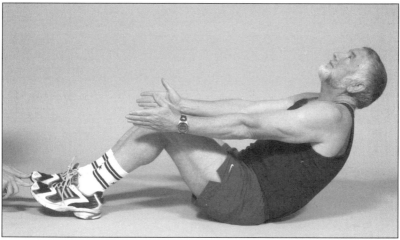

Abdominal exercises: 3 sets of 8 repetitions

Start with your legs bent and your feet pushed up against a wall.

Start with some tension on your stomach muscles by lowering your back a little. This is your starting position.

Breathe in when you go down, curling your back and squeezing your stomach muscles.

Go as low as you can, then breathe out on the way up, squeezing your stomach muscles.

Come back up to the starting position not allowing your stomach muscles to relax.

Tip: to make it harder go lower and keep your eyes on the ceiling. Breathing can be difficult so really focus on breathing in as you go down and out as you come up.

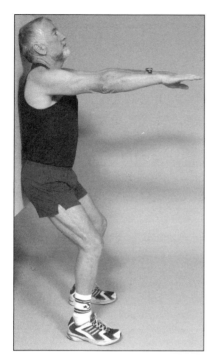 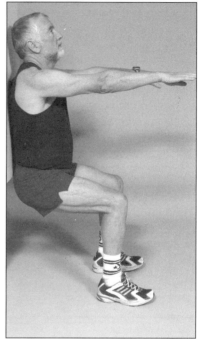

Squats: 3 sets of 8 repetitions

Start with your feet shoulder width apart and your back against a smooth wall or door.

Take your feet away from the wall.

Make sure that your knees do not bend over your toes as you go down.

Hold your arms out for balance.

Breathe in going down (no lower than your thighs parallel to the floor).

Breathe out pushing up, sliding your back up the wall.

Keep your legs slightly bent and repeat the procedure.

Tip: go lower to make it harder. For maximum results keep the tension on your thigh muscles throughout the whole movement.

KEY POINTS

The latest medical research tells us that muscle building through strength training has a very important role to play in fat loss.

Anybody of any age or gender can easily build muscle mass at home without expensive equipment.

Your muscles require energy and the best way to get energy is by burning body fat.

The more muscles you have the more fat you will burn even when you are asleep or sitting in front of the TV.

Greater muscle mass also tones your body.

Strength training has many other medical and psychological benefits.

After a few weeks of muscle building you will feel stronger, trimmer and more energetic.

5

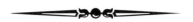

Getting flexible, getting lean and getting in touch with your body

In our modern society, we live very unnatural lives that conspire to make us less flexible and mobile. Very few of us move around as much as we used to. We sit at our desks at work for long periods of time. The recent growth in the number of home computers has made the problem even worse. Computer game addicts like us can easily sit at the computer for hours without moving. We often come home from work and slump in front of the TV. Over the last one hundred years, the population has grown taller, and tall people find it hard to get enough space to stretch and move and tend to suffer more from inflexibility problems.

Why is it important to become more flexible?

There are many advantages of becoming more flexible. These include helping to lose fat, enabling your body to operate much more effectively, keeping you mobile, preventing injuries, helping you do more and get more out of life, and reducing stress.

Fat loss

While many people are aware of the benefits of flexibility, not many fully appreciate the important role that being flexible also plays in fat loss. Stretching and relaxing muscles improves the ability of the body to provide fat as a fuel source to all the working muscles. By increasing blood circulation fat is transported faster and more effectively to the working muscles.

Many men in particular regard regular stretching and relaxing that helps keep us flexible as an optional extra when it comes to fat loss and good health. Yoga classes, for example, tend to be attended mainly by women.   Men may see the benefits of good nutrition, exercise and strength training but flexibility is seen to be somewhat passive and not really important.   But men are generally much less flexible than women (in more ways than one!) and would benefit even more. Being flexible helps fat loss, either directly or indirectly, for both men and women.

Why didn't I get told this ten or twenty years ago? My back and knees have never been better and I have dropped two pant sizes in three months. I need this flexibility to continue my trade as a carpenter.

TONY, HAMILTON HILL

Enables your body to operate much more effectively

One of the main benefits of being flexible is that it helps your body operate more effectively. When you stretch your shoulder, for example, you open up the muscles and tendons allowing your blood to carry rich nutrients to stimulate and strengthen that part of your body. As we said in a previous chapter, an efficient circulatory system will carry fats to your muscles where they are consumed and used for energy. Stretching stimulates the muscles around veins to increase blood flow back to the heart.

Enhanced mobility

Stretching and relaxing exercises are particularly useful for the lower back. It has been said that there are two kinds of people. People who have back problems and people who will get back problems. Not only does a bad back make us feel miserable, but it also stops us getting the great fat loss benefits of moving freely. Proper stretching and relaxing will help prevent back problems. If you already have a serious back problem, you should seek professional help from a physiotherapist or other specialized health professional.

Prevent injuries

Another advantage of stretching is that it prevents injuries particularly if you have been exercising hard or lifting heavy weights. The efficient blood flow that you get from stretching takes away the toxins that accumulates in your muscles. If you exercise hard, you release lactic acid – a form of poison – that makes you stiff and sore the next day. But if you stretch, this lactic acid will be flushed away very quickly enabling you to recover and start exercising again sooner.

When you do strength training exercise you tear tiny muscles, which then regrow to become larger and stronger. But this process also contracts your muscle making them less flexible and more vulnerable to injury. Stretching counters this muscle contraction and makes your muscles long, lean and more efficient and less likely to be damaged. Therefore, stretching and relaxing helps to prevent injury, which means you will not have to take time off your training program.

Helps you do more and get more out of life

If your body is supple through regular stretching, you will be able to enjoy ordinary, everyday activities more such as hanging out the washing, painting the lounge room or throwing a Frisbee with the kids. These pursuits will no longer feel like drudgery and you will burn fat while you are having fun.

Reduce stress

An enormous benefit from stretching and relaxing is that it can reduce your stress levels. Dr Garry Egger, a specialist in the scientific aspects of preventative health, warns about the dangers of long-term chronic stress. Such stress can increase obesity by encouraging the over consumption of high fat snack foods and alcohol. Most of us who have at some stage eaten or drunk too much when we've been stressed can understand only too well what Dr Egger is saying.

In his book, *The Fat Loss Handbook*, Dr Egger maintains that being stressed also makes us feel less in control of our lives and threatens our self-esteem and self-confidence. It is during these stressful times that you are more likely to stop eating well and to stop exercising. It's very tempting to binge on comfort foods or to go to the pub after a hard stressful day and get sloshed. But a few minutes doing simple stretching and breathing exercises will help you relax and cope with the temptation to over-indulge.

Some people who are highly stressed also stop moving. Many highly stressed people sleep much longer than they need. Some hardly ever get out of bed or leave their house. This lack of activity when coupled with an increased intake of food and drink is disastrous. A vicious cycle develops: they gain more body fat, become less fit, lose their self-confidence and their self-esteem plummets. They then turn to more food for comfort.

A big problem with stress is that it can eventually kill you. When we are stressed our body pours adrenalin into the bloodstream to provide us with the energy to either run away or fight, both normal reactions to stress (the 'fight or flight' response). Your body will use adrenalin before burning any fat which is also pumped into your bloodstream. If you exercise, you burn up this fat and there is no health problem. But if you don't do something active, the fat stays in your blood stream and can help to clog your arteries. At the same time, if you are over-stressed - distressed - your heart has to work much harder. Eventually, if you are stressed over a long period of time you may end up having a heart attack or a stroke.

It certainly pays to find ways of reducing stress so that you can continue to lose fat and take pressure off the heart. Stretching and relaxing the muscles is one strategy. Exercising is another. When done properly, stretching, relaxing and exercising will send you into a meditative state where your body and mind become one and you become calm and stress-free.

I used to get home from work tired and stressed and grab a stubby or three. I would then reach for the chips and other snack foods. But now a few minutes of light exercise and stretching calms me down and it's much easier to resist temptation – well most of the time.

EAMON, EAST FREMANTLE

We don't guarantee that either stretching, relaxing or exercising will eliminate all the stress in your life, but it will certainly help. Many of those who have done Ric's program have found that through gaining control of their bodies they are much more able to take control of their lives. A sense of being in control is one of the most powerful ways of turning bad stress (distress) into good stress, which can be very productive. If you are feeling lean, strong and fit, you are much more able to say no to unreasonable demands and not let encounters with unreasonable people become stressful. If you are seriously stressed, there are numerous books you can read, courses you can attend and specialists you can consult.

Ways to become more flexible

There are many ways to become flexible. Later in this chapter Ric will show you seven simple exercises that will give you all the flexibility that you require. The great advantage of Ric's exercises is that you can do them anywhere at any time of the day. You may wish, however, to attend classes that teach you to stretch and relax such as Yoga and Tai Chi, two of the most popular organised ways to help you become more flexible. Both have many other scientifically proven benefits for mind and body. There are other approaches that also work well.

Yoga: the union of body and mind

Yoga has many scientifically proven health benefits. When practised regularly, it promotes relaxation and enhances your sense of well-being. Cardiologist and author Dr Dean Ornish uses Yoga in conjunction with good nutrition and exercise to reverse the build-up of plaque in the coronary arteries of his patients. If you are concerned abut your heart or arteries you might want to consult his book *Dr Dean Ornish's Program for Reversing Heart Disease* which is listed in the Further Reading section.

At first I found stretching and relaxing so boring. I'd much rather go out and run for an hour. But the longer I keep at it the better I feel. My back in particular is so much more flexible.

NADIA, FREMANTLE

Finding the right Yoga teacher is important. Anybody can set up as a Yoga teacher and not all Yoga instructors are properly trained, whilst a few are more interested in making money than in providing a health service. It is wise to ask to see the Yoga teacher's qualifications before joining a class. Yoga exercises are usually conducted in groups, although private instruction is also available. A typical session includes breathing exercises, body postures and meditation. Each Yoga instructor has his/her own style, and classes range from very easy to extremely strenuous. Hatha Yoga is very gentle and relaxing. Iyengar Yoga is more physically challenging. The latest Hollywood craze, Ashtanga Yoga, is extremely demanding and not suitable for the unfit.

It's a good idea not to sign up for an expensive course before you know if it will be the best one for you. To make sure you'll be comfortable with the teacher's approach, ask to observe a class before you sign up or ask if you can try one session before you commit yourself. Also, if you have any doubts about the exercises, stop immediately as you may hurt yourself. Some Yoga teachers, particularly those who teach the more strenuous forms of Yoga, may be overenthusiastic and push you too hard. You should select a program that will leave you rested and relaxed and that you will enjoy.

Tai Chi: a slow dance for health

The ancient Taoist sage Lao Tzu taught that, "it is the stiff old tree that snaps in the strong wind, while the blade of grass bends and lives to see another day". Look at a young sapling bending in a strong breeze and you can appreciate the essence of Tai Chi: developing and maintaining supple strength.

Tai Chi has benefits very similar to Yoga. This traditional Chinese conditioning exercise combines deep breathing, relaxation, and slow, gentle, structured movements. Tai Chi literally means "moving life force" and the activity is like a slow, graceful dance. Tai Chi is based on the Chinese Taoist belief that good health results from balanced chi, or life force. Tai Chi is a particularly safe and effective method of exercise and relaxation for everyone, especially for older adults because it is so very gentle.

Many of the claims about the benefits of Tai Chi have also been substantiated through medical research. This is hardly surprising given that Tai Chi involves both gentle aerobic exercise and strength training, although people may not be aware of this when they are doing it because it seems so easy.

Some people, especially those who are used to very vigorous exercise, may find Tai Chi a bit boring at the start when they are learning the basic movements. But keep at it – as Eamon did – and you will find that it is a wonderful activity that you will both enjoy and get great benefits from for both your body and mind.

During the first few weeks of Tai Chi I wondered what I had got myself into. I found the movements difficult to do and to remember. Then one day something magic happened and it all flowed. I got a real sense of peace and balance and was hooked.
                                    EAMON, EAST FREMANTLE

If you want to learn Tai Chi, contact the Taoist Tai Chi Society of Australia. The society holds numerous classes throughout Australia.

The scientifically proven benefits of both Yoga and Tai Chi if practised regularly include:

➤   Reduced heart rate and lowered blood pressure.
➤   Increased relaxation and concentration.
➤   Strengthened muscles and bones.
➤   Improved balance, flexibility and coordination thus preventing falls.
➤   Improved posture.
➤   Efficient elimination of toxic waste from the body.
➤   Opening the lymph glands in the groin and armpit facilitating the release and elimination of toxins.
➤   Better mental alertness and relaxation of the body and mind - a great way to lower your stress levels.

Flexibility exercises

If you do the following 7 simple exercises regularly, your flexibility, posture and range of movement will improve dramatically.

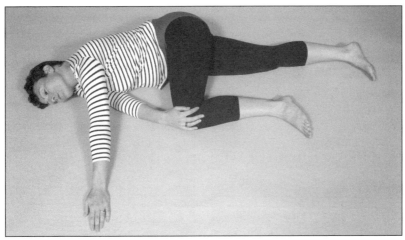

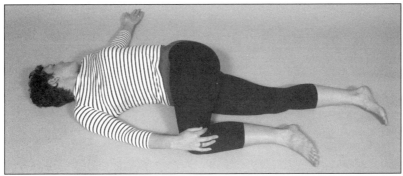

Spinal stretch (hip, lower, middle and upper back, shoulders)

Start by lying on your right side with your left leg bent at 45 degrees.

Place your right hand on your left knee to keep that knee on the ground throughout the whole movement.

Your left arm is straight and parallel to the ground.

Taking a breath in, bring your left arm up to the ceiling.

As you breathe out let your arm go over to the left side, keeping your eyes on the palm of the hand.

It doesn't matter if your arm is a long way from the ground as long as your left knee stays on the ground on the right side.

Keep breathing deeply and with each breath out try to relax all your muscles and let the left arm go lower and lower.

This is a strong stretch so hold it for 30 seconds then breathe in and take your left arm over to the right side.

Release your knee, allow the left leg to straighten and relax onto your back.

Repeat the procedure for the other side.

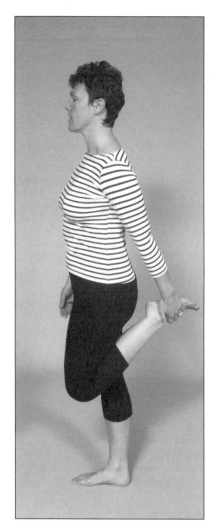
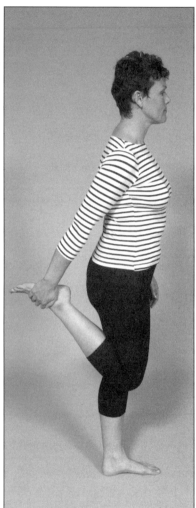

Thigh stretch (front of upper leg)

Stand next to a wall so you can balance on one leg.

Bring your foot up at the back towards your buttock, bending the knee.

Grasp your foot with your hand and bring it further towards your buttock.

Keep your thighs together (if possible).

Breathe deeply and evenly for 20 seconds +.

To make the stretch a little stronger push your foot back into your hand and bend the knee of the leg you are standing on. Keep the thighs together.

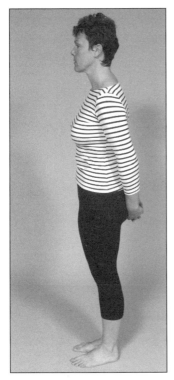 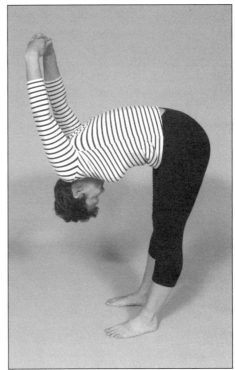

Hamstring and shoulder stretch (back of upper legs, lower back and shoulders)
Start with feet shoulder width apart, toes facing forward, hands linked together at the back with arms straight.
Take a deep breath in.
Start bending forward as you breathe out, keeping the legs straight throughout the whole movement.
Keep the arms relaxed at the back.
Bend as far forward as possible as you continue to breathe out. Do this slowly.
Take another deep breath and when you start to breathe out bring your arms up and over your body, keeping the arms straight.
This is a very strong stretch so don't worry if you can't bend too far or bring your arms up very high.
Keep breathing deeply and evenly and hold this position for 20 seconds **+**.
To make this stretch easier, start with your buttocks against a wall to help support your lower back.
The breathing is really important with this stretch so always work to the sequence above and breathe as deeply and evenly as possible.
When you are ready, lower your arms and bend your knees before coming back up to a standing position.

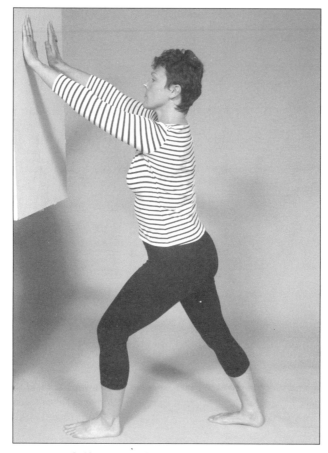

Calf strength (lower leg at the back)

Start with one leg away from the wall, as straight as possible.

Place your hands onto the wall with all of the weight on your back foot.

Take a deep breath.

As you breathe out push back into the heel of your straight leg putting all of your weight on this leg.

Keep your hips in line with your back leg and your back.

Keep pushing into the back heel as you breathe deeply and evenly and hold for 20 seconds.

Bend the back leg slightly but keep the pressure on your heel.

Feel the stretch move down towards your heel in the lower leg. Hold for 10 seconds.

There is no pressure/weight on the front foot.

Inhale and move back into a standing position.

Repeat for the opposite leg.

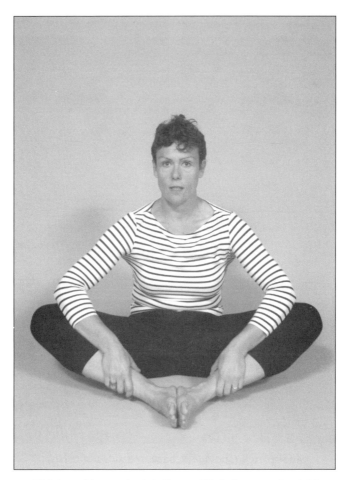

Thigh and knee stretch (inner thigh, knee and pelvis)

Start in a sitting position with your feet together as close to your groin as possible.

Place your elbows on your knees.

Breathe out slowly and push down onto your knees with your elbows, pushing the knees towards the groin.

Keep breathing deeply and evenly, pushing down each time you breathe out and keep the pressure there as you breathe in.

Hold for 20 seconds +.

Inhale and relax back into a sitting position.

To increase the stretch bring your head down towards your toes as far as you can comfortably as you breathe out.

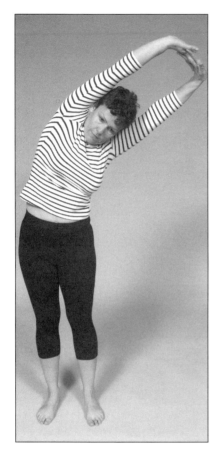 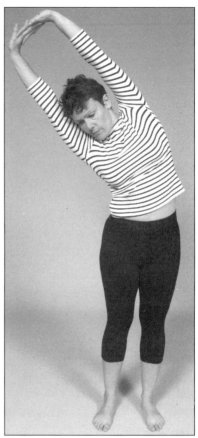

Side stretch (shoulders, back and sides of torso)

Start with feet shoulder width apart, arms as straight as possible, fingers linked with the palms facing the ceiling. Stand straight.

Take a deep breath in and as you start to breathe out lean over to one side keeping your hips straight.

Keep breathing deeply and evenly for 15 seconds then breathe in to go back to a straight position.

Breathe out and repeat movement to the other side, keeping the arms straight the whole time.

Hold for 15 seconds then breathe in as you straighten into a standing position.

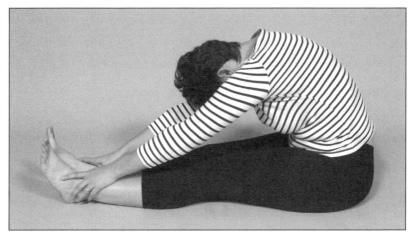

Hamstring stretch (back of thighs, back and neck)

Start with your legs straight out in front of you in a sitting position.

Take a deep breath in and as you breathe out stretch your arms down your legs, keeping the knees flat and straight the whole time.

Once you have fully exhaled, stop. Take another breath in and see if you can breathe out and stretch a little further.

Try to relax your head and neck, feeling the stretch through the back of the legs, the lower, middle and upper back and the neck.

Keep breathing once you have stretched as far as it is comfortable.

Hold for 20 seconds (longer if possible).

Breathe in as you come up, back into a sitting position.

KEY POINTS

Exercises that help you become more flexible will also help you to lose fat.

Being more flexible prevents people from having falls.

Keeping flexible is the secret to staying young.

Stretching and relaxing exercises will greatly benefit your mobility, stress levels and general well being.

Flexibility exercises will also help alleviate or cure many medical conditions.

Flexibility increases co-ordination, muscle strength and tone and reduces recovery time from injury.

Stretching and relaxing exercises, either on your own or in classes such as Yoga and Tai Chi, also help to integrate the body and mind.

6

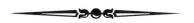

Eight week power program for maximum fat loss and fitness

We wrote this chapter for those of you who are determined to achieve very rapid changes and are ready to make the commitment necessary to achieve these changes. This dramatic fat loss program certainly will not be suited to everyone. You must really want to do this especially as it may involve making major changes to what you eat and what you do. But the benefits will be enormous and well worth the effort. And, of course, you can always adapt the program to suit yourself.

We don't expect that everybody is ready at this stage to make the changes nor is it necessary that everyone do so. You may decide to modify the program if you are not quite ready for such a major change. So if you want to achieve smaller changes more slowly over time, then why not?

We suggest that you read carefully what we have to say below before you make a decision.

This is a demanding program but please note that we are not going to ask you to go hungry or to exercise yourself to exhaustion. Both starvation and exercising too hard would not only be a waste of time but would actually set you back. This program follows the guidelines laid down by leading nutritionists and other health professionals. But if you have any medical problem, you should consider discussing this program with your GP (preferably one who is up-to-date with current nutrition and exercise information) before you start.

A few suggestions before you start

1. Do a little planning beforehand. It is worthwhile writing down the reasons why you want to make a commitment. Put these somewhere so that you can read them regularly, such as on the fridge door.

2. Study the suggested food menu and draw up a shopping list.

3. We strongly urge you to discuss what you are doing with your partner or family. They may be very supportive and a great source of encouragement or they may be unsure or even threatened about what you are trying to do and may tend to sabotage your efforts. Explain that it is only for eight weeks and that you are not expecting them to do what you do.

4. Don't become a 'food nazi' and drive your family and friends nuts.

Most people who follow a program such as this may get self-doubts especially if they have tried other programs and failed. Understanding the reasons why you are doing things will help when you go through these almost inevitable periods of self-doubt. You may, for example, think you are actually getting bigger because of your increased muscle size. But if you realise that as your muscles get bigger you will eventually burn more fat and you'll be leaner and stronger by the end of the eight weeks, then you are more likely to persist. It's worthwhile contacting a health or fitness professional that you trust to keep you motivated and on track during the 8 weeks.

What you can expect for your commitment and efforts

We are all individuals so we can't set absolute figures that apply to everyone but the following are reasonable expectations:

Fat loss

How much fat you lose will depend on how big you are right now. The more fat that you need to lose now and the closer you stick to this program the more spectacular will be the results. Most people reading this book should expect to drop two or more dress or trouser sizes. Please remember not to use weighing scales, as these are an inaccurate and discouraging way to try to measure fat loss. In fact, you may even get heavier initially as you build muscle – this is good! This increase in weight, which usually occurs around the 4-week period, is only temporary.

Greater energy levels

Your energy levels will increase dramatically if you follow the guidelines of eating smaller meals regularly throughout the day. This increase in energy will enable you to follow the exercise program.

Greater fitness

You will notice that you become much fitter. Again, the degree of extra fitness will vary according to the individual and the more unfit you are the more gains you will make. A rough estimation is that your fitness will increase by 30 to 50 percent after just eight weeks on this program.

Enhanced strength and muscle mass

Expect to notice changes after one to two weeks. Your muscle mass will probably increase by about .5 to 1.5 kilos. By increasing your metabolic rate, you can expect to burn up to 800 extra calories each day.

Better skin tone, circulation and general health

You will notice improvements in how you look and how you feel especially if you drink lots of water. Your immune system will be functioning optimally so you are less likely to get colds and flu.

Enhanced sleep quality

You will sleep better but you'll find that you may not need as much sleep because you will fall into the deeply refreshing sleep much easier. As a result, your body will feel much better and regenerate much easier and quicker.

Higher self-esteem and self-confidence

You'll feel much better about yourself and feel more in control as you stick with the program and begin to see the results.

Greater flexibility and range of movement

You'll move more easily after doing the stretching and relaxing exercises. You should see an increase of between 20 to 50 percent after the first few weeks of the program.

Lower blood pressure

If you regularly monitor your blood pressure using a blood pressure monitor, you may find that your blood pressure will decrease the longer you stay on the program. This is more likely to happen if you eliminate all alcohol during the eight weeks.

The power program

The program is a repeat of much of what we have said in the earlier chapters but it is more specific for this intensive program.

Food

Follow the individualised menu plan. Eat five to six small meals a day. Drink lots and lots of water - try to drink 4 litres a day. Combine protein (such as fish etc.), fats (such as avocado etc.) and complex carbohydrates (such as oats etc.) with every meal. Avoid simple carbohydrates, even the healthier ones, for the time being. Therefore, no rice, pasta, bread, cereals, potato, cakes, chocolate, ice cream and so on for the eight weeks.

Strength

Strength train three times a week, about 40 minutes each session, exercising all body parts and muscle groups.
Weeks 1-2: three sets of eight exercises with 10 seconds rest
Weeks 3-4: three sets of ten exercises with 10 seconds rest
Weeks 5-6: three sets of twelve exercises as slowly as possible with a full range of movement.
Weeks 7-8: four sets of eight exercises if possible and slow the movements right down.

Visualise each muscle group the whole time you are working it. The more slowly you go the better the results so it pays to really squeeze. When you feel your muscles burning, you are getting maximum results for effort. Your muscles are broken down as you work hard but within 48 hours rest they will regrow even stronger. So burn, burn, burn!

Cardiovascular fitness

Exercise every day for the eight weeks you'll be on the program. Aim to spend 30 minutes per session. Stay in your training heart rate zone, which is 65 percent of your maximal heart rate. Refer to chapter two if you're unsure of your training heart rate.

Remember that you can do anything that works your heart such as walking, cleaning, shopping, gardening, swimming, flying a kite or sex. Break up the 30 minute sessions into two lots of 15 minutes or three lots of ten minutes if you wish. For example, you might spend 15 minutes walking in the morning and another 15 minutes doing vigorous housework in the evening.

Flexibility

Spend 10 to 15 minutes every day stretching your large muscle groups. Refer to chapter 5 on Getting Flexible. Stretch before and after your cardiovascular exercise. It's just as important to stretch when you do your strength building. You can stretch while watching TV, or in the shower or at work. Relax into the stretch as much as possible. Visualise the muscle stretching and lengthening and always breathe, breathe, breathe.

Remember, this program will last for eight weeks and eight weeks only. This is for rapid, maximum fat loss. After the eight weeks you will be able to go on to a more flexible maintenance program.

The maintenance program

Once you are happy with your fat loss and fitness, you may want to start introducing simple carbohydrates such as heavy grainy bread, potatoes and brown rice if you still crave them. But continue to make complex carbohydrates, proteins and good fats the bulk of your food. You may also wish to cut back on the intensity of the exercise program, but keep up some exercise that you enjoy. Have a day off once a week – a feast day – when you eat whatever you wish. You can also enjoy treats such as chocolate, alcohol or ice-cream more often but combine them with fresh fruit, oats or nuts. Continue to monitor your progress and if you find that you start to put on excess fat again, then return to the power program for a few days. And continue to enjoy feeling healthy, lean and well.

KEY POINTS

Our eight week power program will maximise fat loss.

To succeed, you will need to be clear about your goals and be highly motivated.

The program is an optimal fat loss program and you may decide to achieve results more slowly over a longer period if you wish.

The program draws upon the synergy of good nutrition, cardiovascular fitness, strength training and flexibility for maximum results.

By following the program, you will see rapid gains in how you look and feel, which reflect your body's greater health.

After eight weeks, you go on to a much more flexible maintenance program.

EXAMPLES OF IDEAL DAILY EATING PLAN

BREAKFAST
Porridge and fruit
Home made muesli and low fat milk
Fruit salad and yoghurt and nuts
Omelette with onion and capsicum (alternate vegetables) and fruit
Scrambled eggs with grilled tomato and cheese
Boiled eggs with cheese and fruit (separately)

SNACK
Raw nuts (almonds, cashews)
Fruit (and cheese)
Cheese (and fruit)
Yoghurt and fruit
Boiled egg and tomato (and cheese)
Carrot, celery, capsicum, cucumber sliced (plus dip such as hummus)
Avocado, tomato, cucumber and cheese slices

LUNCH
Chicken and salad (use extra virgin or flaxseed oil for dressing)
Grilled fish and mixed vegetables (mashed, steamed, microwaved etc.)
Bolognaise vegetables and minced meat (low fat)
Tuna or salmon patties (plus vegetables or salad)
Tinned tuna or salmon and tomato salad (plus cheese / avocado)

DINNER
Roast chicken with Greek salad (no oil)
Chicken / pork stir fry (use Braggs Amino Acids)
Grilled fish and vegetables with oven baked potatoes (sweet if possible)
Vegetarian meat loaf (add salad / vegetables)
Beef and vegetable stew (sweet potato instead)
Spinach lasagna (add salad / vegetables if desired)

Exchange lunch / dinner recipes regularly

FRUIT
Kiwifruit, apples, pears, strawberries, cantaloupe, rockmelon, oranges, mandarins, bananas (not many!), watermelon, peaches, apricots, nectarines etc. Best are the fruit in season.

VEGETABLES
Tomatoes (cherry etc), sweet potato, pumpkin (great for carbohydrate!), spinach, broccoli, cauliflower, carrots, zucchini, cucumber, eggplant, onions, capsicum, celery, cabbage, squash, runner beans, snow peas, peas, alfalfa, lettuce, bean shoots, pine nuts etc.

Variation is important with each meal. For example combine five to six veggies rather than two to three.

NUTS
Almonds, brazil, cashews, hazelnut, pecan, peanut, walnut, pistachio

BEANS / PULSES
Lentils (all colours), chick peas, lima, red and kidney beans, etc but not peanuts (not a nut)

OILS
Extra virgin olive, flaxseed oil, Braggs amino acids

7

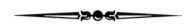

Frequently asked questions

In this chapter we answer the questions that most people ask. We go over many of the most important points that we have made in earlier chapters and introduce some new information.

Why can't I lose fat?

Probably because you don't know how to. You are not eating enough of the right foods and are either not moving enough or are exercising too hard. Many people are also too impatient and if they don't lose lots of fat immediately, they give up eating and exercising sensibly or go on a fad diet that makes them fatter. It's worthwhile getting your thyroid levels checked by your GP as a sluggish thyroid, which is quite common, makes fat loss more difficult. Hormonal problems can also slow down fat loss. For some people there are psychological factors involved and they may need the help of a psychologist or psychiatrist. (Dr Rick Kausman's book, which is listed in the Further Reading section, discusses how to change one's negative attitude toward eating and body image.) Some prescription medicines also make it hard to lose fat. But healthy eating habits and moving around more works for most people if they are patient.

How difficult is it to maintain fat loss?

It's not too difficult to lose some fat but the difficulty is in keeping it off. Over 90% of people who lose fat through dieting eventually put it all back on again. But the very good news is that people who develop their own eating and exercise plans and build them into their lifestyles can keep the fat off.

Can my children follow the same eating program?

Yes. The program is suitable for all ages.

Why does my male partner find it easier to lose fat?

Because males have much more of the hormone testosterone that builds larger muscles and results in a higher metabolism rate that burns fat. On the other hand, women are more aware of the dangers of being over fat and are more likely to do something about it. Women have a further advantage in that they live longer even if they are more over fat than their male partners.

Every time I try to lose fat or get fit my partner or friends try to sabotage me. What can I do?

Unfortunately this happens all too often and there is no easy solution in many cases. (Getting rid of your partner may be too drastic!) Many people, particularly if they are over fat themselves, are threatened when their partner starts to achieve a new slim body. The hard decision you may have to make is whether your right to be fit and well is important to you and then find some way of communicating your need to your partner. Relationship counselling may be a possibility.

Are anti-fat drugs the answer to the 'fat problem'?

No! According to Dr Hakerwell, president of the Victorian Medical Association, there is no such things as a wonder pill for obesity. Some drugs obtained under a doctor's prescription stop you ingesting excess fat and others curb your appetite, but drugs are not a solution by themselves. Drugs work only when used with a healthy diet and exercise. Nutritionist Dr Rosemary Stanton is also critical of anti-fat drugs as a realistic approach to fat loss. They should only be used as a very last resort and under close medical supervision. The same applies to drastic surgical procedures such as wiring one's mouth or stapling one's stomach.

And don't be fooled by glib ads in the media for magic fat burning pills. If you read the fine print, you will see that they must be combined with sensible eating and exercise. There's no scientific evidence that the pills themselves make any difference. If it sounds too good and too easy to be true, then you can be sure it is.

What role does genetics play in body shape and size?

Genetics does play some role so it's important to set realistic fat loss goals. If your parents are both very tall and very thin, then you are likely to have less of a fat problem than your friend with short stocky parents. But your excess fat is determined more by what you eat and how much you move than your genes.

What is the best form of exercise that will help me lose fat?

The best way to lose fat is to use a combination of aerobic exercises, such as walking, and strength training. To burn fat effectively, your body needs a lot of oxygen so for most people walking, or easy jogging, is best. If you are breathing very hard, you are using up too much oxygen and so will burn less fat. Strength training increases your muscle mass, which burns fat even when you are resting. The simple exercises in this book will build your muscle mass but if you are keen you can get excellent results working with a suitable qualified fitness trainer. Tai Chi, Yoga or Pilates can also help build up your fat burning muscles. With about 3 hours of aerobic exercise and 2 - 3 sessions of strength training a week you will get maxmum results, but any exercise will help.

How do I find the time to exercise?

With just half an hour day six days a week (a total of three hours – the equivalent of one night spent in front of the TV) you will make substantial progress. You can build incidental exercise into your day such as walking to the local supermarket. When you get fitter you will have more energy, get more things done and spend less time ill. You will also greatly increase your chances of living longer. You will be less stressed and able to make decisions more quickly, which will save you time and energy. And you'll spend a lot less time visiting doctors.

Am I too old to make changes?

No. You're never too old to get leaner, stronger, more flexible and fitter. Older people are usually more sensible and may have more time to make changes. Many people in their 60s and even older are leaner and fitter than they were in their 30s. Anybody can benefit from weight training, and we all need to maintain our flexibility.

I am not interested in exercise but can I still benefit from the nutritional program alone?

Yes - getting your nutrition right is very important. But you are also much more likely to maintain your fat loss if you incorporate some extra movement into your lifestyle. The very best results are achieved with a combination of good food, sensible exercise, a little strength training and some stretching.

As a woman I am concerned that the weight training will make me too large and bulky. What do you think?

Weight training in fact will make you leaner and smaller. The only way as a woman you can build large muscles is to spend hours and hours in the gym lifting very heavy weights or by taking illegal drugs such as steroids.

Why don't fad diets work?

Most rapid weight loss diets work on reducing weight - not fat - through cutting food intake so low that the body is semi-starved.

You can quite easily lose weight initially, but most of this will be water and valuable muscle. Muscle is very important in burning fat so when you stop dieting you will have more fat but less muscle than when you started. In addition, when you try to lose fat too quickly your body takes defensive action to prevent fat loss. Your body metabolism – the speed at which your body burns fat – will slow down. Your body will also produce more of an enzyme that stores fat. For most people diets are a total disaster. Diets fail also because they become far too boring for most people.

What's wrong with eating lots of bread? Many health authorities recommend that we do.

The carbohydrates in most supermarket bread products have high glycaemic indexes because of the quick processing and baking process. This means that most breads are quickly converted to glucose and then quickly converted to energy. There is also a wide variation among breads. White and wholemeal breads are of little nutritional value. Multigrain brands are better. The best breads are very heavy grainy breads such as soy and linseed. Eat grainy breads and if you want maximum fat loss, consider reducing or cutting them out altogether for a while at least. And consider omitting or reducing butter and margarine and other high fat spreads. Instead use hommous or some other healthier spread.

Why is a pot or beer belly so dangerous to health, especially for men?

Men are more likely to accumulate fat around the gut. Fat stored around the waist is released into the bloodstream at a rate 4-7 times faster than fat around the buttocks and hips, which is where females tend to store it. This excess fat in the gut region acts like mud in a hose blocking off arteries and leading to higher rates of heart disease, diabetes, gallstones and some forms of cancer. A pot belly is now considered the most dangerous form of obesity. The good news is that you lose fat first from the abdomen so it's much easier to shift. Even a few kilos of fat loss could save your life.

What's a fat loss plateau and what can I do about it?

Almost everybody who loses fat at some stage comes to a temporary halt. Often people get discouraged at this stage especially if they have made initial good fat loss progress. The plateau indicates that your body wants to settle at this new level of fat. The important thing to realise is that this is not a failure of you or the program. If you don't put on more fat, you have been successful. If you want to continue your fat loss, you may wish to make some more changes in your nutrition and exercise regimes but don't fall into the trap of panicking and going on a diet. Unfortunately, most people give up just before they start to achieve the very best results. You may consider getting some advice and support from a health professional if you need support. You may also, of course, decide that you are happy with the way that you are at least for the time being.

How do I know that I am losing fat?

A very important question. Being able to monitor your fat loss is a very powerful motivator, but it's very difficult to be objective. It's a good idea to take a photograph of yourself before you start, preferably with the minimum of clothes. You will soon be able to see the difference after a few weeks of sensible eating and exercise. Another way is to use a belt. When you can pull it in a notch you have lost fat. Or check your clothes. If they start to become loose you are doing very well. Health professionals can take your skin fold measurements and there are other more sophisticated tools to measure body fat. Avoid using ordinary weighing scales, which are not an accurate indicator of fat loss. Special scales are now available to help determine how much fat is in your body. When you stand on the scales an undetectable electric current is passed through your body and gives you a measure of your body fat as well as your body weight.

Who is the best person to help me lose fat?

Your GP can advise you about the reasons why you need to reduce fat but may not have the necessary background knowledge in nutrition or exercise physiology. At any rate, GPs seldom have the time necessary to evaluate and to develop an individualised nutrition and exercise program. Increasingly, GPs refer these patients to other health professionals such as dieticians and exercise physiologists. Some of the more reputable health and fitness clubs offer expert advice. Be a good consumer. Learn as much as you can. Talk to people who have achieved long-term changes. It's important to find a health professional with whom you feel comfortable and who can help you achieve your goals safely.

I've heard that people who drink alcohol are healthier than teetotallers? What's your advice?

There is some evidence that people who drink just one or two standard drinks a day have a lower rate of heart disease than those who don't drink at all. On the other hand, individuals who drink heavily are much more likely to suffer from a whole range of health problems. Current medical opinion recommends that if you enjoy one or two drinks a day, don't stop. If you regularly drink heavily, cut back or cut out alcohol altogether. And if you don't drink, don't start just in case you develop an alcohol problem.

Why do people get fatter as they get older?

There is probably no important biological reason for men and women to get fatter as they grow older. The main reason is that older people become less active. Inactivity results in loss of muscle and thus reduces the metabolic rate, which is the rate at which the body burns fat. It is therefore very important and highly beneficial for older people to exercise and maintain muscle strength.

A friend of mine went on one of those high fat diets and lost heaps of weight. What's wrong with that?

Plenty. Most of the weight loss is water and includes lean muscle. When you come off the diet, as almost every body eventually does, you regain the weight and are even fatter because you have lost fat burning muscle. Over 90% of people who lose weight through dieting eventually put it on again and often with more fat. Very high fat diets, such as the Atkins Diet, can also cause dehydration, headaches, light-headedness, irritability, bad breath, constipation and kidney problems. These diets can lead to heart disease and can be fatal in individuals with diabetes. For the vast majority of people the only way to lose fat and to maintain fat loss permanently is to make long term changes in their lifestyle.

What about very low fat diets?

It's true that most people eat too many of the wrong fats found in biscuits, cakes, takeaway foods and processed foods. But reducing or eliminating bad fats does not mean that you should eliminate all fats. You need some fats that are found in good oils, such as extra virgin olive oil and fish. Some research conducted by cardiologist Dr Dean Ornish (see Further Reading) suggests that a very low fat diet, like the Pritikin Diet, can help people with heart disease, but other research also suggests that healthy people can be harmed by a diet that is very low in fats. Consult your GP before you make a decision.

What's the glycaemic index and is it useful to help me lose fat?

The glycaemic index ranks foods according to their effect on blood sugar levels. Foods with a low glycemic index release sugars into the blood more slowly. Foods with a low glycaemic index are therefore more satisfying, so you're less likely to feel hungry. For example natural muesli and All Bran (low glyacemic index) are a much better choice than toasted muesli or Coco Pops (high glycaemic index). The glycaemic index of white and wholemeal bread is around 70, multi-grain is much better with 42, while soy/linseed is better still with a low 19. People with diabetes are urged to have diets based on a low glycaemic index that can help them to control their blood sugar levels. But just because a food has a low glycaemic index doesn't mean that it's low in saturated (bad) fats or low in calories. Unfortunately, foods like ice cream, cakes, and chocolate, all have a low glycaemic index but can still make you fat. There are plenty of books on the glycaemic index which you may find useful particularly if you have diabetes. But most people do not need to know about the glycaemic index and may in fact become confused.

My husband is over fat and snores a lot. Is this a problem?

Unfortunately it is. Heavy snoring is usually due to excess fat in the tongue and neck. Besides being very irritating, heavy snoring can help cause high blood pressure and heart disease. Both the snorer and his partner wake up feeling fatigued and irritable. The cure is simple: lose fat.

Are vegetarians healthier than meat eaters?

Usually yes. For example, one study found that vegetarian 7th Day Adventists had only one fifth the hypertension of meat eating Mormons. But it's not just diet. Generally, vegetarians tend to be more active, to drink alcohol sensibly and not to smoke. There's no medical reason to become a vegetarian. Fish, for instance, is extremely healthy. Vegetarians, especially women, can develop low iron levels unless they are careful. An extremely healthy diet includes plenty of fish, perhaps a very small amount of lean meat (for iron and vitamin B12), chicken, preferably free range, and lots of fresh fruit and vegetables.

What are free radicals and antioxidants?

Free radicals are produced naturally when your body uses oxygen. Free radicals are also caused by smoking, too much alcohol, and pollution - even too much exercise. They attack body cells which may lead to premature ageing, cancers, heart disease, arthritis, and by destroying brain cells may result in Parkinson's and Alzheimer's Diseases. Antioxidants are potential lifesavers. They mop up the free radicals and neutralise them. Where to find them? Surprise! Mainly in vegetables and fruit! Eat a wide variety of different coloured vegetables and fruit so that you get the full range of antioxidants. If you are exercising hard, then you need even more.

I'm going to a great party next week. There will be lots of good food and wine. What should I do?

Enjoy yourself! One day of indulgence a week will make no difference in the long run. In fact, it's a good idea to have a day a week when you eat and drink what you like.

FURTHER READING

We have consulted numerous books and articles that relate to nutrition and fitness. Many popular books on fat loss and exercise are useless, if not misleading and even dangerous, including some written by health professionals.

We strongly recommend the following books and articles because we have checked the authors' credentials and the information they have provided which is based on scientific research. Always keep in mind that new research is happening all the time. Our list includes books that will appeal to the general reader as well as those that are more suitable for health professionals.

Aston, Donna *Body Business.* Viking, 2001.
Donna Aston is a highly experienced personal trainer who has represented Australia at the Ms Universe body shaping competition. A very balanced and sensible approach to good nutrition and effective exercise. Her recommendations on why we need to eliminate highly processed food are particularly insightful.

Egger, Garry & Binns, Andrew *The Experts' Weight Loss guide for doctors, health professions ... and to all those serious about their health*. Allen and Unwin, 2001.
A slightly misleading title as this book is aimed mainly at general practitioners. It reviews the latest literature. Dr Egger is Scientific Director of Gutbusters waist loss program. Dr Binns is a general practitioner who specialises in treating patients with obesity.

Egger, Garry and Swinburn, Boyd *The Fat Loss Handbook A Guide for Professionals.* Allen & Unwin, 1996.
Provides detailed scientific evidence for fat loss and exercise programs. This excellent book is essential reading for all health

professionals interested in obesity and fitness. Each chapter has a comprehensive reference list. The bible for health professionals!

Egger, Garry & Stanton, Rosemary *GutBuster 2, The High Energy Guide*. Allen & Unwin, 1995.
Although written primarily for men, this well written guide to waist loss by two of Australia's most respected nutritionists and researchers is also very useful for women.

Kausman, Dr Rick *If Not Dieting, Then What?* Allen & Unwin, 1998.
An excellent book for people, especially women, who feel bad about their bodies. A medical practitioner who specialises in weight management, Kausman discusses the important issue of how to avoid the psychological and emotional risks of obsessive dieting. He emphasises the importance of enjoying food and feeling good about oneself. He shows how the diet industry and the media exploit women's negative body image.

Nelson, Miriam E. *Strong Women Stay Slim*. Thomas C. Lothian, 1998.
An excellent well researched and written book by an American medical researcher. Her advice is aimed primarily at women but is also applicable to men.

Nelson, Miriam E. *Strong Women Stay Young*. Thomas C. Lothian, 1997.
Nelson's companion book on strength training is also based on the author's extensive scientific research and medical training. Her program is also suitable for men.

Ornish, Dean *Dr. Dean Ornish's Program for Reversing Heart Disease The scientifically proven system to reverse heart disease without drugs or surgery.* Random House, 1990.
According to Dr Ornish, a cardiologist whose research has been published in high quality medical journals, his nutrition program can reverse serious medical conditions, particularly heart disease. Some critics say that his very low fat vegetarian diet may not be suitable for healthy people.

Robbins, John *The Food Revolution How Your Diet Can Help Save Your Life and Our World.* Conari Press, 2001.
A very detailed, compelling and at times provocative account of the health advantages of a vegetarian diet and the moral question of the cruel way that the meat industry treats animals. Robbins draws upon extensive published research to attack popular unhealthy fad diets such as *Dr Atkin's New Diet Revolution, Enter the Zone,* and *Eat Right for Your Blood Type.* However, he ignores the health advantages of fish.

Stanton, Rosemary *The Diet Dilemma.* Allen & Unwin, 1991.
Australia's best-known nutritionist, Stanton exposes the many scams and rip-offs in Australia's lucrative diet business. Highly recommended.

Ric Isaac's *Fit for Health*

Would you like help and support in putting into practice the fat loss and fitness programs discussed in this book?

Ric Isaac's *Fit for Health* provides:
- personalised eating plans
- exercise classes for fat loss and fitness
- personal training
- Yoga classes
- massage
- reflexology

All of Ric's services are provided in a safe, friendly and supportive environment.

For further information:
Phone: 0411 220 600
Email: ric_isaac@hotmail.com

10 Wray Avenue
Fremantle
Western Australia

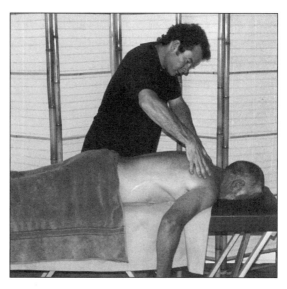